An Edgar Cayce Health Anthology

Selections from
The A.R.E. Journal

A.R.E.® Press • Virginia Beach • Virginia

A Note to the Reader

The A.R.E. does not present any of the information in this book as prescription for the treatment of disease. Application of medical information found in the Cayce readings should be undertaken only under supervision of a physician.

More in-depth information on certain medical problems is available to A.R.E. members in the Circulating Files. For information on the Files or for a list of suppliers of items found in the Cayce readings write to: Membership Services, A.R.E., Box 595, Virginia Beach, VA 23451.

2nd Printing, June 1982

3rd Printing, November 1983

4th Printing, November 1985

Printed in the U.S.A.

CONTENTS

FOREWORD

Because of the demand for health-related information based on the Edgar Cayce readings, we were encouraged to make available under one cover a collection of such writings. In reviewing the contents of *The A.R.E. Journal* from its inception in 1966 to the present, we had in mind to choose a wide variety of preventive, curative and health maintenance themes.

The selections in this anthology are primarily feature articles. In addition, because of their popularity and utility, we included a selection of "shorts" from Dr. William McGarey's *Medical Research Bulletin.** The MRBs appear interspersed between the feature articles.

In the table of contents, titles of articles appear in capital letters, while MRBs appear in upper and lower case to help you distinguish one from the other. The index should also prove useful in locating topics.

Good health to you!

Editorial Staff
of the A.R.E.

---

*The *Medical Research Bulletin* is published by the A.R.E. Clinic, Inc., in Phoenix, Arizona, as a communication medium for physicians and others in allied health service and healing fields.

GEARING THE BODY FOR THE AQUARIAN AGE

by Lawrence M. Steinhart

Most of us are aware of the psychic evolution coming about in the Aquarian Age, and many of us are increasingly aware of the spiritual promises which are unfolding in the human race. However, few of us are taking practical steps toward preparing our bodies, the vehicles through which we have earthly expressions, for the changes that are also to come in the physical world. It is within the body, the temple of the living God, that we must meet God face to face.

The sleeping Cayce, as sages before him, advised seeking the way within oneself. "It is *within* that there is the kingdom of heaven!" (877-27) According to the readings, the man Jesus—who became the Christ—was and is a pattern of the way in which man can develop to his ultimate purpose.

Lifetime after lifetime man wonders, "What is my ultimate purpose?" Pursuing the answer to this question he evolves, but in that evolvement makes some mistakes. Often the same mistake is made repeatedly. Recurring habit patterns build what might be termed the "karmic chain," a whole series of related mistakes. One's own habits are difficult to recognize; knowing oneself can be a painful experience, but necessary for the evolution to the next level of consciousness. Enslaved by our karmic chains, we seek to break out via the weakest link, which for many of us is the appetite.

Diet

The readings frequently recommended that one should eat foods grown or produced in the vicinity in which the individual resides. In this way he could acclimatize himself to the vibrations of the area. In today's world of polluted, synthesized and unnatural foods, Cayce's words are especially valid. Foods which ripen naturally and are eaten where they are grown are

1

always preferable to exotic luxuries shipped from "far-away places with strange-sounding names." For, as the readings stated:

Shipped vegetables are never very good.   2-14

Have *most* of the foods that are grown in the area where the body lives, as much as practical.   337-27

Use fruits, nuts, berries of all natures or characters that are grown in the environ of the body . . .   1771-3

. . . plenty of both raw and well-cooked vegetables, and those that are grown the more in the environ in which the body finds self.   2066-2

This is a good reason to sprout beans and seeds at home, because not only are sprouts high in vitamins and minerals, but also they are the most easily digested form of vegetable protein. Absolutely fresh from the sprouter, their vitality is undiminished. One-half cup of sprouted soybeans contains the same amount of vitamin C as six glasses of orange juice.

Most people know that cooking vegetables lessens their vitamin and mineral value. Despite the glamor of the jet-age kitchen (microwave ovens, teflon-coated pans and instant frozen gourmet dishes), eating cooked food is still second best. However, if we *must* cook it, we might consider preparing it in cooking parchment (Patapar paper was referred to in the readings), in its own natural juices. This has the Cayce seal of approval as has the pressure cooker:

Q-14. Consider also the steam pressure for cooking foods quickly. Would it be recommended and does it destroy any of the precious vitamins of the vegetables and fruits?
A-14. Rather preserves than destroys.   462-14

We would include the Jerusalem artichoke in the diet . . . cooked in its own juices—that is, in Patapar paper, so that all the juice of same may be stirred or mixed with the bulk when this is eaten.   243-36

. . . the preferable way to prepare [the vegetable] juices would be through cooking the vegetables after tying them in Patapar paper; not putting them in water to boil, but cooking either in the Patapar paper or in a steam steamer, so that only the juices from the vegetables may be obtained—and no water added in the cooking at all . . .

A little later the body may begin with stewed chicken, or broiled chicken or broiled fish . . . [Even] the chicken or fish would be better cooked in the Patapar paper or a steam cooker.
133-4

People are waking up to the fact that aluminum changes the chemistry of certain foods prepared in it. More and more we are switching to stainless steel, enamel and porcelain pots. We are using steamers for our vegetables so that the vitamin content doesn't run down the drain. But Cayce's recommendation for the use of a cooking parchment is still the method which delivers the greater amount of nutriments. This is not a complicated affair, and it is also economical as the parchment can be used over and over again.

The readings further suggest that condiments should be used *after* the cooking of foods.

The cooking of condiments, even salt, *destroys* much of the vitamins of foods.
906-1

The regular use of gelatin was advised. It was suggested that raw vegetables and salads be prepared in a gelatin mold, making sure that none of the juices escape. Because gelatin is obtained from animal cartilage, vegetarians may prefer to use Agar Agar flakes, which are derived from seaweed. It is not the vitamin content in the gelatin itself which is so important but rather its acting as a catalyst.

Q-4. Please explain the vitamin content of gelatin. There is no reference to vitamin content on the package.

A-4. It isn't the vitamin content but it is ability to work with the activities of the glands, causing the glands to take from that absorbed or digested the vitamins that would not be active if there is not sufficient gelatin in the body. See, there may be mixed with any chemical that which makes the rest of the system susceptible or able to call from the system that needed. It becomes then, as it were, "sensitive" to conditions. Without it there is not that sensitivity.
849-75

Red meat is to be eaten rarely (excuse the pun!); the meats preferred in the readings are lamb, poultry and fish. They explain that, unless one is extremely active and able to "work off" the energy created by the red meat, the excess would act as a dross in the system.

In the diet keep away from red meats, ham, or rare steak or roasts. Rather use fish, fowl and lamb . . .   3596-1

And in the matter of the diet, keep away from too much greases or too much of any foods cooked in quantities of grease—whether it be the fat of hog, sheep, beef or fowl! But rather use the *lean* portions and those that will make for body-building forces throughout. Fish and fowl are the preferable meats. No raw meat, and very little ever of hog meat. Only bacon [crisp]. Do not use bacon or fats in cooking the vegetables, for this body; for these tend to add to distresses in those directions of this segregation and breaking of cellular forces throughout the system.   303-11

Keep away from heavy foods. Use those which are body building, as beef juice, beef broth, liver, fish, lamb, all may be taken but never fried foods.   5269-1

It is known that the amino acids in protein are the essential nourishing factor. The flesh itself is not digestible and therefore remains in the system as dross. Perhaps the most important reason for limiting the intake of red meat is that we take on the vibrational pattern of everything we eat. The readings advised against eating pork because it has the lowest vibrational pattern of any meat.

In this world of coffee and carbonated drinks, the drinking of water—*aqua pura*—is not as widely practiced as good health requires.

Q-12. How much water should I drink daily?
A-12. From six to eight tumblers full.   574-1

The readings further stated that foods taken into the body would act in a more beneficial manner if a glass of water was taken before a meal and one just after. The following reading also suggested the drinking of half to three-quarters of a glass of *warm* water immediately upon arising as a way to clarify the system of poisons.

. . . for, as has oft been given, when any food value *enters* the stomach *immediately* the stomach becomes a storehouse, or a medicine chest that may create all the elements necessary for proper digestion within the system. If this *first* is acted upon by aqua pura, the reactions are more near normal.   311-4

These dietary suggestions can be habits easily acquired, and once acquired are performed involuntarily, leaving the mind free for greater things.

Mind Is the Builder

For in the beginning God moved and mind . . . came into being—and the earth and the fullness thereof became the result of same.   5000-1

The mind governs the body more or less; consequently, the mind should dwell on beautiful things if we would have a healthy body.   87-1

"Mind is the builder." This statement, repeated throughout the readings again and again, is a subject for study in itself. Nobody will doubt the power of the mind, but are we prepared to attribute to it the myriad daily mishaps and unwanted patterns of behavior in our lives? Patterns which *could* be changed by the conscious changing of mental attitudes. Are we prepared to trace many—if not all—of our sickness to attitudes? Should we wish to research this subject, we each have a perfect guinea pig nearer to us than our right hand—ourself.

We can start working on changing some of the more obvious mental patterns first, such as exchanging anger for patience. Anger is itself a sickness of the brain giving rise to many more sicknesses, while patience is something we came into this three-dimensional plane to learn. Patience is not long-suffering, though that is part of the experience, too; patience is the joyful acceptance of being. Let us ascertain that our love for those close to us is true love, with no trace of possessive love—this eliminates jealousy. It makes the object of our love feel less like a "thing" and more like a person. Working on these mind twisters individually, one should find one's life changing. Sickness will become less a part of the pattern as harmony enters.

Eliminations

Seekers after the causes and cures of the many ills which rack the human frame find that the physical readings very often zeroed in on the colon. It has been pinpointed as the hotbed of disease and the breeding ground of microscopic monsters more hideous than have ever been created by the "horror specialists" in Hollywood. However, the elimination of poisons through the alimentary canal is a subject usually discussed between mothers and children under five years of age, after which time it is expected that an entity should be well enough versed in the complicated eliminatory processes of the body to be able to fend for itself. The readings unequivocally state that the body should have at least one complete evacuation each day and if this is not accomplished naturally, we should aid the process.

... there should never be allowed a twenty-four hour period without an evacuation. For this, as indicated, makes for an accumulation of toxic poisons or drosses that tend to make for pressures upon the nervous system, in the sympathetics or the vagus and the cardiac centers, and an engorgement and an enlargement of the heart's activity. Hence the colonic irrigations. Hence the better activities in the food values, rather than such a conglomeration as to make for distressing conditions. Hence, also, the constructive mental activities in regard to same.   294-184

Q-4. Should anything be taken for eliminations?
A-4. Correct better by the diet than by taking eliminants, when possible. If not possible to correct otherwise, take an eliminant but [alternate] between one time a vegetable laxative and the next time a mineral eliminant.   3381-1

Q-2. What laxative is best for this body?
A-2. There should be no one individual laxative. Rather vary from oils to sodas ...   294-184

The use of the enema with a saline solution is perhaps the easiest method. Other methods include eliminants of many types: broken doses of olive oil, abdominal massages with same, castor oil packs and, for almost everybody, an internal wash (colonic) occasionally. The readings explained that just as we wash the body externally we should also wash it internally. For this they recommended saline/soda, Glyco-Thymoline and other solutions of an alkaline nature, used at body temperature. They stated that if the specific instructions were followed, it would be good for the body and would bring a more natural functioning, strengthening the walls of the colon and encouraging its muscular activity (peristalsis).

The colon is the main artery of the eliminating system. If it is obstructed in its function, the other systems of elimination must help to carry the burden. A strong body odor is evidence of toxins being expelled by the perspiratory system while halitosis is the result of the respiratory system taking on an extra job. Skin problems are the manifestation of some irregularity in the eliminating processes and to seek a camouflage for these symptoms will only *temporarily* disguise the fact that the body's functioning is off balance. It is unfortunate that people brag that they "never perspire, even on the hottest days." Perhaps if they did, their aches and pains would be less apparent. To release toxins from the system through perspiration is one of nature's ways of cleansing the system and it is frightening to see millions of dollars spent on advertising campaigns that sell products designed to stem this flow.

. . . those things that have been as a stoppage for the respiratory activity [have] in part affected the *emunctory* circulation, and . . . made the tendency for conditions in the superficial circulation that are unsatisfactory.   563-4

Deodorant/anti-perspirants are available and offered for use not only for the underarm area but also for the groin area. When asked what ingredients in such preparations were harmful, Cayce stated: "Anything that closes the pores of the skin to prevent perspiration." (2072-6)

Q-11. Should one use a deodorant, especially under the arms, to stop perspiration . . . ?
A-11. The *best* to use—the safest—is soap and water!
                                                                        404-8

Adjustments and Massage
The solutions offered for physical disharmonies were varied. In a survey of the treatments suggested by the readings, mechanical adjustments—through osteopathy and chiropractic—were the most numerous. The correct alignment of the spine allows the body to rally its own healing forces. The readings promised that the body contains within itself all that is necessary for our perfect healing and resuscitation, providing faulty eliminations do not hinder.

These adjustments are merely to attune the centers of the

body with the coordinating forces of [the] cerebrospinal and sympathetic system. Thus the body is purified or attuned so that it in itself and nature does the healing.   3384-2

These [osteopathic treatments] are beneficial—whether once a week, once in ten days, twice a month, ten times a year, or forty times a year. When needed, take them!   1710-10

Massage plays an important part in the coordination of the various tasks that the body has to perform, and the oils and combination of oils recommended as the medium include an infinite variety from Russian White Oil to peanut oil.

Dream Guidance
Where can we turn for guidance? For those of us whose meditations have not yet reached the level of receiving visions, guidance can be sought through dreams, the interpretation of which was given as a most important facet of spiritual growth.

. . . dreams, in whatever character they may come, are the reflection, either of physical condition . . . or of the subconscious, with the conditions relating to the physical body and its action . . .   294-15

Dreams can give us the answers to questions which are in the foreground of our daily lives, despite the fact that they may not have surfaced in the conscious mind. Sometimes we are not ready to accept dream advice, in which case symbols reoccur in various guises until we actually do something about the advice. Anything which might interfere with our harmonious existence rises to the surface of our dreams to be worked out. When we work with our dreams we have an ally which can work with us, side by side, in meeting the opportunities which confront us daily. Dreams may help us make the decisions which will keep us in tune with the world around us. Ignoring our dreams is tantamount to enrolling in college and not attending the lectures. Dream interpretation is an aid which is becoming more widely researched and practiced in the Aquarian Age.

The Spiritual Path
The readings gave as the basic premise of life that the Lord our God is *One*. Our bodies contain in their three-part unity all

that is to be found in the universe. It is no wonder, then, that every realized man has exhorted us to seek the truth within ourselves.

This is the spiritual goal achieved by meditation, or seeking to attune ourselves with God. It is the putting aside of our earthly self and practicing the art of "being." Where, then, is one to start? How can one become a part of the Aquarian Age and fit into its pattern, a pattern which is moving towards a world as yet seen only in a dream-like stage? If we are to allow the Cayce readings to guide us, we will begin immediately with that which sings to us the most sweetly. When one piece of the puzzle fits into the picture of life, the movement has been started. Waiting will not make it happen; applying the necessary daily disciplines will. After the first step has been taken, whether in the physical, mental or spiritual, we are on the path.

Folk Medicine . . . Using That in Hand

Grape juice was suggested in the Cayce material for many reasons. It has a type of sugar in it, apparently, that does not metabolize in such a way that it makes one obese. Thus, we suggest for those patients who want to lose weight that they drink four ounces of a mixture (half-and-half) of grape juice and water prior to each meal. This satisfies the appetite to some extent and may be beneficial for the intestinal tract.

However, when grape juice is carried a bit further in the processing, it becomes wine. One of our patients, who is now in her sixties, tells us a story about wine unlike any that we've heard before. As a two-year-old, Lucy could not walk nor stand without assistance. We don't know exactly what her diagnosis was, but it was potentially permanently disabling and certainly had something to do with a congenital hip deformity. Her mother apparently heard from someone that hot red wine applied to the extremities was what the child needed. She applied hot compresses—hot wine poultices—to her daughter's legs, thighs and hips every day for a year. I checked her legs recently and they are as straight and solid as any I've seen. Her mother used what was at hand, and healing followed.

THE BENEFICIAL EFFECTS OF MEDITATION

by George Hollins, Jr., M.D.

Some may wonder how a doctor could know much about meditation, and I admit I know considerably more about medication than I do about meditation, though I'm in the process of learning.

For many years I attended a church whose minister gave some very inspiring sermons which usually ended with the admonition that we ought to change ourselves and change our lives. I noticed that he never gave any suggestions as to how we should do it, although I remember he sometimes said that we should begin at home.

There were a number of things about myself that I thought needed changing, but I didn't know how to go about it. I had an inner feeling that there was more to be learned, so I kept on searching. In a public library I found some books on Zen, but these didn't seem to be what I was looking for. At last I was led to read a book that said you could change yourself by meditation and what's more, you could also find union with God by meditation, although some other things were required, too. This book was *Autobiography of a Yogi* by Paramahansa Yogananda. There were lessons available from the Self-Realization Fellowship which he founded, and I took these. Soon after this, I mentioned my interest to a friend who told me about Edgar Cayce and the A.R.E. I began coming to the meditation retreats at their Virginia Beach headquarters. I also went to the S.R.F. Headquarters in California several times, and took the Kriya Yoga initiation there. This is an ancient meditation technique that was revived about a hundred years ago by Yogananda's guru's guru's guru, Babaji.

My purpose is not only to stimulate an interest in meditation, but also to inspire perseverance and persistence in daily practice. One must continue to meditate even though there seem to be no immediate results for months or even years. I think I expected results too soon, but as time went on I realized that the final goal was a long way off and that meditation was a progressive process of consciousness expansion. I found that there were also progressive benefits to be gained from its practice, and they were physical, mental and spiritual. These benefits are by no means confined to oneself, because meditation can and should be used for others.

The physical benefits can affect ourselves and others. This frequently, but not always, involves prayer. Probably most of you know what I first learned through reading the books of Emmet Fox; that one of the secrets of effective prayer is to first raise the consciousness as high as possible. This can be done to some degree by reading one of the Psalms over and over, or by chanting, but it can be done even better by meditation. It may not be necessary to use any words in prayer at all, but just silently visualize the person to be healed and see him surrounded by light and love, filled with peace and joy.

Some of you may have heard of Silent Unity, where there is a prayer room which is open twenty-four hours a day to receive requests for help from people all over the world. Last fall I had an opportunity to spend a week at a retreat at Unity Village. While there I heard Wilma Powell, one of the supervisors of the program, tell how they obtained such good results from prayer. She said that they go into a state of meditation, which they call entering the silence. She described this as a feeling of light or well-being, and said that from this state of elevated consciousness they send out their prayers.

The Cayce readings have this to say about the physical benefits of meditation:

... life in its activity is the expression of the divine influence in a material world. And individuals in the application of that that comes in their ken of activity may, through the drawing wholly, solely, upon the Creative Forces within, *change* their own surroundings, their *own* vibrations, within their bodies!
404-3

Know that all healing forces must be within, *not* without! The applications from without are to create within a coordinating mental and spiritual force.   **1196-7**

For all healing, mental or material, is attuning each atom of

11

the body, each reflex of the brain forces, to the awareness of the Divine that lies within each atom, each cell of the body.

3384-2

. . . let's analyze healing for the moment, to those that must consciously—as this body—see and reason, see a material demonstration, *occasionally* at least! Each atomic force of a physical body is made up of its units of positive and negative forces, that brings it into a *material* plane. These are of the ether, or atomic forces, being electrical in nature as they enter into a material basis, or become *matter* in its ability to take on or throw off. So, as a *group* may raise the atomic vibrations that make for those positive forces as bring divine forces in action into a material plane; those that are destructive are broken down by the raising of that vibration! That's *material,* see? This is *done* through *Creative* Forces, which are God in manifestation!

281-3

This sounds rather technical, but I think Edgar Cayce was saying that all matter is structured, or undergirded, by divine energy or divine force. This is what we can influence by meditation, and, in turn, this can influence material manifestations.

It has been my personal experience to have seen some occasions of spiritual healing. I do not feel that I have yet unfolded to the stage of being a channel for direct spiritual healing except in one or two cases, which were psychosomatic in origin and lasted for only a short time; yet there certainly have been many instances of inner guidance for healing by outer means. One of the most dramatic examples was in the case of a fine elderly gentleman from the Eastern Shore, whom I saw a few months ago. He had a tremendous bone tumor growing from his femur, the upper end of the thigh bone. This had become infected and was causing him severe pain. I put him in the hospital and did a biopsy, which is to take a piece of tissue and send it to the laboratory for study and analysis. The report came back—low-grade malignancy. The orthodox, or conventional, treatment for such a thing as that is to amputate—not only the leg, but the entire pelvis on that side.

In such cases, we doctors don't like to take the whole responsibility on ourselves, so we seek consultation, not only for advice but also for assistance in surgery. My consultant, a young general surgeon, felt that the orthodox treatment was one that should be done, but because of the patient's age I had grave doubts that he would be able to live through such an extensive procedure. The ideal treatment would be to remove the tumor from the leg, but the tumor was of such tremendous size, and was so high up that I would not be able to get a tourniquet on above it to control the bleeding. I feared severe or fatal hemorrhage, irreparable damage to the main artery to the leg, or extension of the infection into the muscles of the thigh.

The pathologist assured me that the tumor was one that would recur only locally, and slowly at that. As time went on it became more and more imperative to do something. I turned to meditation and the Cosmic Beloved for help. In a little while a response came as an unconventional plan unfolded before my closed eyes. The key to this plan was to have the general surgical consultant make an incision up in the abdomen and put a temporary clamp on the main artery to the leg, while I made an incision in a different way from the one I had originally planned. I would then suspend the leg after surgery with the thigh straight up, so that the drainage would be down and away from the muscle.

I discussed this plan with my partner who was going to assist me, and at first he thought it would work. The consultant still thought the orthodox treatment was better, although he finally agreed to go along with the role I planned for him, which was to clamp the main artery. The hardest part came the day before surgery was scheduled. My partner told me that he doubted that we could get the tumor out through the incision because of its huge size. (This illustrates one of the reasons why it is a good idea to keep your inner guidance to yourself because your friends are likely to talk you out of it.) In this case, because teamwork was so essential, I couldn't keep it a secret, but I did keep the source of my idea secret. I held to my inner conviction and we went ahead with the operation. Everything worked out beautifully, and afterward all three doctors (another partner helped) told me how glad they were that it had been done the way it had.

When it comes to healing self, for the most part my personal experience has been in the form of guidance to a medical solution. However, last fall I had an experience of being healed of an attack of bronchitis during a group meditation, with one of the members acting as a channel. Coughing, which had been keeping me awake night after night, and which had not responded to antibiotics or cough syrup, subsided completely and did not return.

Besides healing self and others, there are sometimes

situations in life which need healing. I have made a daily habit of asking a blessing during meditation on my home, on my office, going on from there to the whole Tidewater area, and then the planet Earth and all those who dwell on it. The effect on my home is subject to interpretation. So far I have not observed any remarkable effect on the planet, but I really believe that this blessing has had an effect on my office. In an office with five doctors and fourteen women, you can imagine that there are sometimes moments which are not too harmonious, although it has been almost miraculous how these women get along together. If one of them seems to be stirring up negativity, it isn't long before she finds a job more to her liking somewhere else, or her Navy husband gets transferred, or some other reason comes up for her to leave. Also, when someone leaves on short notice an even better replacement shows up before the last moment. One time a new partner turned in his resignation shortly after our senior partner had retired, and we were all up to our ears in work. Nevertheless, our differences were settled amicably and the resignation was withdrawn.

Another important physical effect is security. In the *Bhagavad-Gita* Krishna declares that even a little meditation will save us from dire suffering in this world. One of the members of my meditation group put this a little differently when she said she had noticed that when she doesn't meditate regularly, things don't seem to go too well. This seems to illustrate what is called grace. When we meditate regularly we live under grace, which I believe is what the 91st Psalm refers to as "the secret place of the Most High." Emmet Fox wrote that many people have been helped out of all sorts of trouble by repeating this Psalm over and over again, until they raise their consciousness to a level higher than their trouble. After all, raising your consciousness is the same as meditation.

Perhaps the list of physical benefits of meditation should also include supply—if not of actual wealth, at least of life's necessities. Jesus said, "Seek ye first the kingdom of Heaven and all these things will be added unto you." Surely the kingdom of Heaven means a higher state of consciousness, or Christ Consciousness. Perhaps these words mean that we actually have to find this state before things are added, but I think they mean what they say—that if we are seeking, or are in the process of seeking, they will be added. This includes health and prosperity.

Another physical result that I have found is that I have less fatigue in doing the day's duties. I find since I began meditating regularly that even in the busiest moments of the day I can pause a moment and feel an inflowing of energy and vibrations such as I feel during meditation, which banishes fatigue.

In working out this outline of physical benefits, I found it difficult to separate them from the mental and spiritual, because they are all so interrelated.

The mental benefits are also for others as well as for self. One benefit for others is healing of mental conditions, and in my personal experience I have found this to be easier than healing physical conditions. For example, I have a patient, now a dear friend, who was so fearful of hospitals and doctors that for months she refused to have a necessary operation for a bone graft to a fracture in the arm. When she finally stopped resisting and went to the hospital, she was so fearful that I dreaded taking her to surgery as much as she dreaded going. However, in meditation the next morning I felt guided to hold her in the light, mentally, and to see her surrounded by light and love, and filled with peace and joy. After that she seemed completely changed and went through the operation without any trouble. During her convalescence she lapsed many times into her old attitudes of hopelessness, despair and anxiety, and even after she left the hospital she used to call me frequently. I would ask her to come to the office the next day, and in the meantime I would meditate and send her these vibrations of light and so on. When she came to the office she would already appear brighter. As the healing progressed, these attacks became less frequent, but even now, when I am in a particularly good meditation I will beam her some more light.

With regular meditation we become easier to live with at home. Our domestic relations with our family or spouse may have been good or not good, but in either case they tend to get better, and I can attest to this personally. A word of caution is necessary here. It is vitally important to keep what you are doing to yourself and not try to convert others in your family; let any change in them take place as a result of your example.

One of the best mental results for both ourselves and for others is better control of thoughts, feelings, and attitudes. Freedom from anxiety and worry is something I have experienced most of all. Why worry when you can turn over all the problems to the Infinite in meditation? When we place ourselves, our loved ones, and all our affairs in the hands of the

Father, we can expect all to be in divine order and for our own highest good.

There also seems to be improvement in attitudes. Resentment, anger, impatience and irritability recede as the peace we find in meditation is carried over into our daily lives. I can truthfully say that I am much happier now than I was before I began meditating. Little things that used to rob me of my peace of mind no longer seem important, when I can turn inward to the serenity and little fountain of joy in meditation.

Another advantage is that when you meditate regularly you tend to know things you should know. Some years ago there was an article on ESP published in, of all places, *The Wall Street Journal,* a paper which I have purchased not more than three times in the last ten years. One day I felt a desire to pick up a copy at a drugstore, and later on in the week, when someone asked me about the article on ESP, I was able to discuss it. I don't have much time to read newspapers, but when there is something vitally important that I should know, I seem to see it or someone tells me about it.

Another improvement has been in memory. I'm sure I'm not alone in having difficulties remembering names of people, books, and things, especially as I get older. I find that often a name which I cannot recall in ordinary consciousness will easily come to mind in meditation.

Then there is the help in creative writing. Many times when I have to compose a paper, or talk on some subject, a key phrase or phrases will pop into my mind during meditation.

There is also the inner assurance that all will go well that is found in meditation, especially before a journey, whether by automobile or jet, or in my case, before a difficult surgical operation. In my experience, I feel this assurance when I ask for a blessing for a safe trip or a successful operation.

The spiritual consequences can also be divided into those chiefly for others and those chiefly for oneself. It must be kept in mind that if I seem to weigh these benefits heavily on the side of the individual, it is because any individual who does not have much spiritual growth himself cannot be of much help to others. It depends on one's use of the benefits received. For example, while one is in an elevated or expanded state of consciousness, one can send out blessings to other individuals or groups of people. I feel sure that this can assist individuals spiritually, and I feel that it would probably help all people on earth if enough joined together in such an effort.

Recently I had the firsthand experience of feeling the long-distance transmission of what—for lack of a better name—I will call vibrations. This seems to be a kind of subtle energy or force, which may be the same thing as Divine Love, and which can be sensed as a joyous feeling of energy, light, and well-being welling up in one. Incidentally, I also learned that, like all good, if we send it out to others we leave room for more to come to ourselves. Not long ago our small Thursday night meditation group was joined by a new member, and I began to notice that I was aware of these same vibrations when she attended, but when she didn't attend I didn't notice it so much. I later asked her about this and she admitted that she had been consciously sending out these vibrations to others in the group. Soon after this she had to take a trip to another state, about a thousand miles away, and was gone for a period of two weeks. At the meeting on Thursday night, I felt the same vibrations as before, but the next week I felt none. When she came back I asked her if she had meditated at the same time on Thursday night as we had. She said she did so on the first Thursday night, but circumstances prevented her meditating the second Thursday. You may say that this was coincidence, but I mention it to show the possibility for sending blessings over great distances to others.

There is still another way that meditation can be of spiritual aid to others and that is through a spiritual law: When we grow spiritually we lift up those around us.

Although I disclaim any pretensions to spiritual advancement, for many are more spiritually advanced than I, I do feel that I have been doing some catching up, and am not as far behind as I was before I started meditating. One of the first effects for me was an increasing inner serenity, found in meditation, and which can be continued into the day's activities. This peace is really God making contact with us, or meeting us as Edgar Cayce put it, in this reading on meditation:

There is that access, then, that way, to the Throne of grace, of mercy, of peace, of understanding, within thine own self. For He hath promised to meet thee in thine own temple, in thine own body, through thine own mind . . . And then enter into the holy of holies, within thine own consciousness; turn within; see what has prompted thee. And He has promised to meet thee there. And there *shall* it be *told* thee from within the steps thou shouldst take day by day, step by step. Not that some great exploit, some great manner of change should come within thine body, thine mind, but line upon line, precept upon precept, here a little, there a little. For it is, as He has given, not the knowledge alone but the practical application—in thine daily experience with thy fellow man—that counts.

922-1

"In the end, the reward is well worth the effort expended. Most of us waste hours each day when just a few moments spent in daily search within would bring more peace and joy, and more true happiness, than any physical activity."

A Search for God, Book II, p. 131

Yogananda, in the poetic language of the East, spoke of the need to keep our inner peace while the storms of life's trials howl and shriek around us. He also spoke of the little geysers of joy that shoot up from within.

Another spiritual outcome is development of psychic powers, such as telepathy, clairvoyance and out-of-body travel. Yogananda said that we should not seek psychic powers for their own sake, but that they would come as we grow spiritually. He illustrated this with a story about a man in India who spent most of his life developing the power to walk on water. One day he met a holy man who told him that he had been wasting his time learning to walk across the river when he could have hired a boatman to take him across for a few cents, and that he should have devoted his life to searching for God alone.

For some time I have made a practice in meditation to ask for a blessing if I am going to perform an operation that day. If all is going to go unusually well, I feel a response of a joyous feeling before the operation. If it was just to be average, I would feel good about it, but would not have the joyous feeling. I will always remember one time when I had a serious case, but I did not have that good feeling. Toward the close of the operation the patient's heart stopped. It was only by the quick action of all members of the operating room staff, using cardiac massage and artificial respiration, that the patient was brought back to life.

This also seems to work for taking journeys. One time I didn't have this assurance when I asked for a blessing before I took my family on an automobile trip. On the way back that night we had a narrow escape from a bad accident, when a car without lights was stopped across the road in our lane and I was partially blinded by the lights of another approaching car.

I've also noticed that for about two years I haven't had to use an alarm clock. I have yet to be late on account of this, although sometimes I've really had to hurry, for I still have the temptation to go back to sleep after waking up. This seems to work best when I put a definite time into the subconscious. Sometimes I'll wake up and look at the clock once or twice ahead of time, but many times it's right on the minute. There seems to be a feeling of compelling urgency to look at the clock if I wake up at the time. It seems to be more than just a built-in timer, because last winter at a medical meeting I was attending there was a paper late in the afternoon that I wanted to hear, but I had time for about an hour's nap in my hotel room beforehand. The paper was scheduled for 4:20, and I felt chagrined when I awoke and looked at the clock and it said 4:20. Although it took me ten minutes to dress and wait for the elevator, I still arrived on time to hear the whole paper. Here it appears that the subconscious not only knew the time, but it also knew the progress going on down in the lecture hall below!

Meditation also is helpful in self-purification, or purgation, if you like, such as eliminating or reducing negative attitudes, thoughts and feelings and substituting for them kind, loving thoughts. This change also includes reduction of personal ego which can be said to be the soul in a state of delusion, or *maya,* as they say in the East. We can feel that we are working more and more for God and less and less for ourselves.

In addition there is an increasing awareness that only the life of the spirit is real and all else is delusion. We can grasp the fact that we are not the body, and not the mind, but something beyond these, when in meditation we can observe the body and the mind and their activities from a higher level of consciousness. We also realize that we are all one when in meditation, and especially in group meditation, we can feel an expansion of ourselves to include other members of the group. This seems to be like an invisible substance that flows out to enfold all the others around.

In my experience, the most wonderful meditation benefit of all is help in practicing the presence of God and in the establishment of a personal relationship with God as One whom we can contact at any time and not just during meditation. We can then truly say with St. Paul, "In Him we live and move and have our being." We can know Him as the Cosmic Beloved Friend to whom we can turn with our gratitude, as well as with our problems. We can feel we have a counselor and teacher who will see that we get the needed experience at just the right time in line with our development.

How can we help but feel a growing love for God when in deep meditation we can feel the infinite and unconditional love He has for us? If I had received nothing else in return for the eleven years I have spent in meditation, an experience I had two or three years ago would have made it all worthwhile. This, too, was in a group meditation. I can say that I was definitely conscious of being in the presence of the Father. It was personal, yet no form was seen and no voice was heard, just a presence. There was a consciousness of an absolutely uncritical, unconditional, all-forgiving love, even though He knew all my faults, all my weaknesses, and all my secrets. It was total, complete love, without reservation. With this was an awareness that His will for me was only good and whatever I experienced in life was for my highest good and soul's growth. Although this is not new, to experience it oneself has a profound effect on one's life.

When we practice this presence of God and personal relationship with God, we can expect His help at all times, not just during meditation. This can be useful, for example, in making important decisions. If we pray deeply and ask for guidance, the Infinite will see that we get it. The answer may come in the form of an inner voice in meditation or by a mental picture. On the other hand, the answer may come in the form of something we see in print during the day's activities, such as something that I read recently which just fitted in with a business decision that I was trying to make. The guidance may be something that someone, even a child, tells you. The Infinite can use many channels to tell us what we need to know.

Meditation helps reduce our karma and helps bring about eventual freedom from the wheel of incarnations by final merging of our individual wave in the ocean of spirit. I like a Hindu chant quoted by Yogananda: "Oh, my saint, wake, yet wake. You did not meditate, you did not concentrate, and passed thy time in idle words. Oh, my saint, wake, yet wake. Death will be at thy door, and you won't have time any more to redeem thy soul. Oh, my saint, wake, yet wake."

I like to think, as the author of this chant apparently thought, that we are all student saints and although we may have many lifetimes of classes ahead of us, and we may fail our courses from time to time, our graduation must come sometime. When that time comes depends on us.

PHYSIOTHERAPY IN THE EDGAR CAYCE READINGS
The Concept of Wholeness

by Mary Alice Duncan, P.T.

A first look at the Edgar Cayce physical readings can be a confusing experience to the professional in the healing arts and to the layman alike. The professional, steeped in his academic training, may scoff at the suggestions given. The average layman is confused by his very lack of knowledge of the anatomy and physiology of the body.

To bridge this gap so that both the layman and the professional may be able to study any of the nearly 9,000 physical readings with greater understanding, one concept above all others—*the concept of wholeness*—needs to be understood. Indeed, until the concept of wholeness has become an integral part of one's own thought pattern, it is almost impossible to understand any of the physical readings.

The Cayce readings did not look at a person as being one-third physical, one-third mental, and one-third spiritual—as if these three parts of an entity were distinct and had to be treated separately, as is often done in standard medical practice. Instead, the readings saw the entity as a *whole* with its various parts, organs, systems, glands, fluids and essences totally and completely *interrelating in their life and function.*

The entranced Cayce simply could not see or consider the physical without the mental or without the spiritual because they cannot be separated; in a sense they *interpenetrate* and they are *one.* The following excerpt which ties God and the physical body together indicates that this interrelationship has existed from the beginning:

For, when the earth was brought into existence or into time and space, all the elements that are *without* man may be found in the *living* human body. Hence these in coordination, as we see in nature, as we see in the air, as we see in the fire or in the earth, makes the soul, body and mind *one* coordinating factor with the universal creative energy we call God.   557-3

The concept of wholeness should be considered even down to the cellular level. Each cell can be thought of as a universe in itself. The readings looked upon the cell as having a consciousness of its own and as having a memory of what its proper function should be. The implication is that each cell has both a mental body and a physical body, and that spirit works *through* the mental body and *in* the physical body of that cell. Recent biophysical research of the RNA and DNA molecules seems to substantiate the Cayce material in respect to the memory function.

The Edgar Cayce records viewed health as a state in which all parts of an entity were functioning in *balance* and in *cooperation* with all other parts. The term usually used for this was *coordination*. The readings did not conceive of illness as just a distortion of a part or a cell or a system. Instead, the bodily distortion was looked upon as an *effect* of illness, not the illness *per se*. Illness was explained as an imbalance *between* parts or cells or systems of the whole entity. The term usually used for this was *incoordination*. The implication is very simply that health is coordination and ill health is incoordination.

It has always seemed to me that if a basic truth is really true in the philosophical sense, then it must also be true if considered from the purely physical. This means that truth is truth from any angle and if it falls short from any viewpoint, then it wasn't the ultimate truth in the first place. In reading 1472-3 the "sleeping" seer said, ". . . Truth is *Truth, ever*—in *whatever stage,* in whatever realm of evolution, in *whatever* realm ye find same . . ." and again in 5030-1 we find, "Truth is truth everywhere the same, under every circumstance." With this as a guideline we might ask ourselves how the concept of wholeness, which is implicit in the physical readings, fits in with ultimate Truth in the philosophical sense.

The answer was given in 1933 when Group One asked the entranced Edgar Cayce for some basic statements of fundamental truth. After first chiding them for not getting this information *themselves* by correlating various statements he had previously given them, he complied with their request by giving them a dissertation on the *Oneness of All Force*. Although the complete reading is commendable and worthy of close study, only a portion can be given here as directly applicable to this discussion.

The basis, then: "Know, O Israel, (Know, O People) the Lord thy God is one!"
From this premise we would reason that: In the manifestation of all power, force, motion, vibration, that which impels, that which detracts, is in its essence of *one* force, one source, in its elemental form . . .
God, the first cause, the first principle, the first movement, *is!* That's the beginning! That is, that was, that ever shall be!
The following of those sources, forces, activities that are in accord with the creative force or first cause—its laws, then—is to be one with the source, or equal with yet separate from that first cause . . .
In the beginning there was the force of attraction and the force that repelled. Hence, in man's consciousness he becomes aware of what is known as the atomic or cellular form of movement about which there becomes nebulous activity. And this is the lowest form (as man would designate) that's in active forces in his experience. Yet this very movement that separates the forces in atomic influence *is* the first cause, or the manifestation of that called God in the material plane! . . .
Hence, as man applies himself—or uses that of which he becomes conscious in the realm of activity, and gives or places the credit . . . in the correct sphere or realm he becomes conscious of that union of force with the infinite with the finite force.
Hence, in the . . . fruits of the spirit . . . does man become aware of the infinite penetrating, or interpenetrating the activities of all forces of matter . . .   262-52

The practitioner of one of the healing arts who is also a student of the Cayce material can hardly fail to conclude that the concept of *wholeness* and the concept of *oneness of all force* are in reality the same. Thus it follows that Edgar Cayce tapped a source of knowledge that was consistent at all levels of understanding—physical, mental, and spiritual.
Perhaps the ability which Edgar Cayce demonstrated could be likened to the operation of an electron microscope, because he actually saw inside individual cells of a living human body. This is what is meant when we say that the readings look at the body at a cellular or atomic level. This ability seems fantastic enough, but, in addition, Mr. Cayce demonstrated something the electron microscope cannot do. He could see the *function* of the cell in relation to the function of all other parts of the

entity—physical, mental, and spiritual. We might postulate that some day science will invent a device to do what Edgar Cayce did. But if that day ever comes, will that super electron microscope deliver sermons of the quality that we find in the data he left?

An intensive study of this information indicates that the concept of wholeness or oneness is actually the foundation stone upon which all other concepts are based. It can be seen undergirding the acknowledgment of psychosomatic illness, in which the readings were far ahead of their time. It underlies the concern for prevention of illness which is so often neglected by present-day therapeutic practice. It accounts for the insistence upon treating the cause of illness rather than just the effect. It is even basic to the understanding of individual differences.

Classification of Physiotherapy Techniques

Throughout these psychic discourses the term *physiotherapy* was consistently used rather than the term *physical therapy.* Because there are people who may be under the impression that these two terms represent a difference in emphasis regarding therapy, it should be noted that the terms are synonymous. At the present time, physiotherapy is the preferred term in Canada and in England; whereas the preferred term in the United States is physical therapy. The training is essentially the same and the various modalities and techniques are the same. However, during most of the forty-three years that the readings were being given, the terms *physiotherapy* and *physiotherapist* were in general use in the United States. Inasmuch as the information generally suggested to "use that in hand," it would appear that the readings followed their own advice even in regard to terminology.

Transcripts in the A.R.E. library show prescriptions recommending virtually every technique normally used in the profession of physiotherapy except such things as ultrasound, which did not come into therapeutic use until a few years after Edgar Cayce terminated his unusual career. Six major classifications of "drugless therapy" were advocated. All but one were and are used in the practice of physical therapy.

Under the broad classification of *electrotherapy,* the readings made use of the modalities of shortwave diathermy, long-wave diathermy, ultraviolet light therapy, violet ray (which is a form of static electricity), heat lamps, and various techniques of low-volt therapy. In addition, they prescribed several devices of which no one had ever heard or used before, such as the wet-cell appliance and the radio-active appliance. These devices were used to bring nutritional and medicinal substances into the body vibratorily.

Hydrotherapy included numerous techniques used to cleanse the body both externally and internally. The most common ways to use water or steam for cleansing were steam baths, fume baths, and colonic irrigations. Concerning the rationale of such treatments, statements were explicit:

. . . hydrotherapy and massage are preventive as well as curative measures. For the cleansing of the system allows the body-forces themselves to function normally, and thus eliminate poisons, congestions and conditions that would become acute through the body.   257-254

Packs of all sorts were advocated to combine the therapeutic benefits of heat itself with purported medicinal effects of the medium used to produce physiological improvements within the body. A partial list of the types of packs suggested includes epsom salt packs, salt and vinegar packs, grape packs, and castor oil packs. Although the precise understanding of how these packs actually effected changes within the body is not known, considerable empirical evidence exists that they are of benefit.

Exercise was suggested often, with both general and specific advice as to its use and rationale for either preventive or therapeutic effects. The most usual recommendation was for walking—done consistently—as the best all-around exercise for most bodies.

Massage was suggested as a specific treatment more than any other one technique. Occasionally massage was the *only* treatment recommended, but more often it was used in conjunction with other measures—particularly with some form of hydrotherapy. There was hardly a major disease in which massage was not one of the recommendations. It was suggested for everything from callouses to head colds and from baldness to muscular dystrophy.

Spinal manipulation was recommended numerous times as an important therapy for selected patients. These techniques have not been a part of the profession of physical therapy in the past as has manipulation of other joints. However, considerable interest in spinal manipulation is beginning to be shown in this country among physical therapists.

Massage as Therapy

Historically, massage is one of the earliest forms of treatment for bodily ills. It has been specifically advocated from the time of Hippocrates up to our present day. Massage is usually done with the hands, although various mechanical devices are sometimes used. Massage manipulations are applied to the soft tissues in order to produce effects on the muscles themselves and also on the circulation of the blood and lymph and on the nervous system.

Massage, like the other broad classifications of drugless therapy, is not exclusively a technique of the physiotherapist, but may be used by a practitioner of any of the therapeutic disciplines. The readings were sometimes specific about who should do the massage and often named both the discipline and the individual.

Occasionally, however, massage by a professional was specifically *not* advised. Instead, the recommendation was that the treatment should be given by a member of the family—one who *loves* the patient. This was so in the case of a seven-year-old girl who had a birth injury resulting in paralysis, loss of vision, deafness, and the inability to speak. She had been given up by the medical profession as hopeless. This case is interesting because it noted that, "This is the bungle of the doctor, not of this soul-entity." (3117-1) The reading did not dwell at length on the physical pathology that was present but preferred to encourage the parents:

True, there are adhesions, and there is the lack of the circulation through portions of the brain. But this is at the beginning of a cycle for body change. Each atom may be changed within seven years. If there are those interested in contributing to this, *begin*. If you are not interested in doing it for fourteen, don't commence! 3117-1

The advice was then given that only the applications of prayer, the wet-cell appliance, and massage were needed. After outlining precise instructions for the wet-cell, it was indicated that the time when the appliance was attached to the body should be "the hour of prayer and meditation." Specific massage information followed:

The massage should be given immediately following the use of the appliance, and must be very carefully administered, very persistently—always away from the head. Use only

peanut oil. Begin with the very first cervical, gently, massaging on each side of each segment, downward, even to the toe tips, along each side of the spine—especially the left side of the body.   3117-1

The parents apparently followed the instructions to the best of their ability but after one year they had a check reading in which they asked if the massage were being done properly. The answer followed:

This is very good, except sometimes you hurry through too quickly. Remember, these are to be given very prayerfully; seeing, feeling, knowing that they are contributing to the general welfare of the body.   3117-2

The next question indicated that the parents recognized that the *direction* of the massage movements was contrary to that usually given, and they asked if the "general regular massage" should be given. The answer was graphic:

When it is necessary or better to massage in other directions, we will indicate it. Here we [have] the tendency, as we have indicated, for a flow toward [the] head. Keep it in that way in which there is a flowing away from the head. If you were to dam a stream, would you sometimes attempt to knock it away so the water could clear a little bit? Not much you wouldn't, if you wanted to prevent it from flowing back! This is just a practical condition that exists in the law of nature itself. Massage away from the head, as we have given. There are areas, as outlined, where the massage may be in a circular motion. It may all be of the circular nature if it will be away from the head always.   3117-2

Perhaps the mother of the child had become pregnant or was ill, because the third question asked, "Due to the mother's condition, for the next few months may the massage be given later than the treatment [wet-cell appliance], by the father when he comes home?":

The massage may be done by anyone who is patient and persistent, but as indicated, do not attempt to delegate to someone else that which should be the privilege and the opportunity of the parents. Others may do it, even a little bit better, yet in mind, in body, in spirit, those who are to heal themselves in healing this body must do the applying.

                          3117-2

It should be noted that the above case was very specific regarding *how* the massage should be done, *when* it should be done, *who* should do it, and *what* oil should be used. Not all readings were that specific; some were just as specific although every detail of the instruction was just the opposite from what [3117] required. This difference illustrates the principle that massage needs to be tailored to fit the individual, which necessitates a close look at the rationale of massage.

A reading given for a 47-year-old woman with minimal pathology had some general comments concerning the regular or general massage which is often termed "Swedish massage":

Massage applications are excellent for each body, and well for this ...

Once in ten days or once in two weeks. This should be sufficient, with the regular activities that the body has ...

... Swedish massage ... is for the superficial circulation, to keep attunement as it were between the superficial circulation or the lymph and the exterior portion with the activities of the body. These treatments should not be hurried, and there should be given sufficient period for the reaction to the body.
1158-11

In the majority of cases, massage was given to improve the superficial circulation and lymphatic drainage as noted above. The following reading given for an 18-year-old boy with leukemia speaks of this and indicates an additional benefit to the nervous system:

The "why" of the massage should be considered: Inactivity causes many of those portions along the spine from which impulses are received to the various organs to be lax, or taut, or to allow some to receive greater impulse than others. The massage aids the ganglia to receive impulse from nerve forces as it aids circulation through the various portions of the organism.
2456-4

The scope of this paper precludes a description of the various massage movements which are used by professionals. The readings appeared to understand these, although the direction of the massage movements was sometimes seemingly reversed from that ordinarily used. However, once certain principles are understood, there is seen to be no conflict with the usual practice of massage.

Massage for the purpose of increasing venous return of blood to the heart or to decrease edema (swelling due to excessive accumulation of fluid in the tissues) should start with the hands placed on the proximal part of an extremity. A gentle squeezing motion is applied to the muscle with the force exerted *toward* the heart. The hands are then lightly moved distally a few inches below where the previous motion started. Then the squeezing motion is applied again with pressure toward the heart. This process is repeated with a rhythmical and constant rate until the therapist's hands are working at the most distal portion of the extremity. In this way, although the motion is downward from the shoulder to the fingers and from the hip to the toes, the *force* of the motion is always toward the heart. When a deep massage is indicated, this technique should be employed because a proper massage should never interfere with venous return. In order to reflexly stimulate the nervous sytem, a very light stroking can be given from proximal to distal (hip to toes and shoulder to fingers) as was indicated in the reading for [3117] quoted above.

One other massage movement advocated often was deep circular friction over scar tissue. This is a technique long employed by physiotherapists. The unique thing about the readings in respect to scars was the use of the combination of camphorated oil, dissolved lanolin, and peanut oil as the massage medium. With persistence in the use of this formula, the successful results of this treatment are often almost beyond belief.

Massage Oils

The Cayce readings implied that the oils used in massage were *absorbed* by the skin and that they acted as food for the underlying structures. This concept is particularly interesting because, until quite recently, the medical-scientific community has rejected the idea that the skin can absorb substances placed on it. In 1964 the report of a clear, colorless, and almost odorless liquid known as dimethyl sulfoxide (DMSO) gave dramatic verification to the premise that the skin is not impervious. DMSO could be painted on the skin of some distal portion of the body and very quickly, having been absorbed into the blood stream, it would be tasted in the mouth of the recipient who would emit a garlic odor on the breath. Finally, the DMSO was excreted via the kidneys.

Although the experience with DMSO does not offer conclusive proof that other substances have the same membrane penetration ability, the possibility can be admitted.

Perhaps research will provide the answer as to whether there is *actual* penetration of the oils Cayce recommended, or whether the penetration is of a *vibratory* nature only.

The readings usually gave a simple formula for the oils to be used in massage. Often plain peanut oil was recommended. And just as often simple combinations such as peanut oil and olive oil; or peanut, olive, and lanolin were advised. In cases where peanut oil alone was prescribed, it was noted that if itching or other skin irritations should occur, lanolin might be added.

Peanut oil is relatively inexpensive and readily available in most grocery stores. Although there is no record of comment about the brand of peanut oil to be used, the experience of A.R.E. therapists, osteopaths, and others suggests that it might be better to use the more expensive, cold-pressed peanut oil which is available only in health food stores. The latter is of a lighter consistency and more absorbable by the body. Because it has no preservative, it is less irritative, but it *must* be refrigerated—allowing the portion to be used to warm to room temperature prior to application.

Occasionally a complicated formula of many different exotic oils was advised as the massage medium. Reading 2302-1 is informative because it contrasts the use of a "special rub" with the exotic oils to the use of a simple lotion for a general massage. The 68-year-old man for whom these readings were given had numerous physical problems including toxemia, debilitation, abscessed teeth, neuritis, and blindness. He was first directed, among other things, to have a blanket sweat or fume bath "to remove poisons from the system," after which his wife was to sponge off his body and then:

. . . massage deeply and heavily along the cerebrospinal system, from the base of the brain to the end of the spine, on either side of the spine, with an equal combination of olive oil and peanut oil. This does not mean just rubbing it on, but massaging it into the system in a circular motion; finding each segment, as it were, along the cerebrospinal system. 2302-1

In the third reading for this same man, he was instructed to keep all of the previous applications including the peanut and olive oil massage, but in addition:

. . . we would compound a specific rub to be used *after* the fume baths—now.

To 2 ounces of Russian White Oil, or Nujol, as the base, add—in the order named:

Cedar Wood Oil	½ ounce
Pine Needle Oil	½ ounce
Peanut Oil	1 ounce
Sassafras Root Oil	¼ ounce
Oil of Mustard	20 drops

These, to be sure, will tend to separate; but before using shake well together, pouring a small quantity in a saucer. Dip the fingers into same and massage along the spine from about the middle of the back *upward* to the base of the brain. Then massage in a circular motion on each side of the spine, each segment and along each side, *downward* to the central portion of the spine . . .

This will stimulate the activities of the optic forces, and we should soon begin to see some light . . .

. . . *this* as given is a special rub, you see, and is only to the 9th dorsal—or from the 9th dorsal to the base of the brain; while the other [peanut and olive oil massage] is over most of the body, you see, as a stimulation to the whole of the respiratory and perspiratory system.   2302-3

Unfortunately, the reasons were seldom spelled out as to why certain oils were recommended in one case and other oils were suggested in another. However, in the case of a 34-year-old female with neurasthenia the rationale for the use of the massage oils *was* given. She was asked to have a massage each night before bed with equal parts olive oil, tincture of myrrh, and sassafras oil. The reading specified how and where the massage was to be administered, and required that it be preceded by moist heat packs to the back:

The activity of the olive oil is as *food* that may be absorbed by the lymph and emunctories of the system, provided the pores and the exterior portions of the body have been relaxed or opened before this is massaged into the system. The activity of those properties as go *with* same, the myrrh and those of the sassafras oil, these add to the *strength* of the muscular tissue, of the sinew along the system, as to carry—the one stimulating the muscular forces, the other carrying to the cartilaginous forces, and to every nerve fiber itself, that of strength and activity.   5423-1

Concepts of Healing

There are those today, just as in Edgar Cayce's day, who tend to discover in his readings a gold mine of magic remedies.

Nothing could be further from the truth. There is *no* magic in the Cayce readings! Every single suggestion made demanded *effort* on the part of the patient, and *effort* on the part of those who worked with the patient—either as doctors, therapists, or family.

Furthermore, the readings *stressed* that the applications do not heal; *the body heals itself.* Apparently the applications, whether colonic irrigations or vitamin supplements or castor oil packs, serve to balance the body so that the forces already *in* the body can accomplish the healing. In the case of a seriously ill 12-year-old girl who had a total of seventeen readings in the course of five months, the parents were repeatedly reminded of these facts:

> It should be known by those that wait and labor and work with the body, the applications in any form for disorders do not *make* life—they only may prepare the way through which life itself *may* manifest.   632-2

> For all forces of health-giving properties must come from *Life* itself—GOD! and the applications are only making for the ability for that spiritual influence to manifest in a material way and manner.   632-5

> For, in *any* application that may be made of *any* nature for healing to a body, it is only to supply that means, that channel through which life energies in a body may find the better channel for manifestation. *Healing* is done by the body. Those applications to same only prepare the way for same to be accomplished.   632-6

In the life reading of a 28-year-old osteopath who had been a physician in a previous life in Caesarea, the statement was made that, "Disease has changed little—their names, their classifications, much!" (2002-1) Yet, the readings didn't seem to speak in terms of disease *per se.* They spoke in terms of *function* and tended to be reluctant even to give names to the various illnesses that were encountered in the course of the physical readings.

Time after time the insistence appears that there is every force in the body for healing and that the body itself has a capability for normal function. One patient was informed that:

> . . . there is in each body, as in this body, those necessary influences to produce body-sustenance and body rebuilding—

if the activities of the glands and organs are made to coordinate. 2769-1

And another patient was told:

... there is every force in the body to recreate its own self—if the various portions of the system are coordinating and cooperating one with another. 1158-11

In most instances where applications of treatment were advised there was the additional suggestion that persistency and consistency of application were necessary. However, usually the treatments suggested were to be taken regularly for a time and then the body was to be given a rest period before repeating the series. This cyclic pattern was to prevent the body from becoming too dependent on the treatments for its activity.

Perhaps the most important advice for physical healing related the physical and mental body to its spiritual source. Here it appears in a conclusive way:

For the law of the Lord is perfect, it converteth the soul. It should be used, not abused, in the application. For unless one makes the application (as the entity found through that experience, as Elias), healing of the physical without the change in the mental and spiritual aspects brings little real help to the individuals in the end. 4016-1

In this material plane, understanding of the physical body and the maintenance of its health is of prime importance in the achievement of wholeness in the spiritual life.

BIBLIOGRAPHY
1. Beard, Gertrude, and Elizabeth C. Wood, *Massage: Principles and Techniques,* Philadelphia & London, W.B. Saunders Co., 1964.
2. Jacob, Stanley W., "DMSO: Potential Usefulness in Physical Therapy," *Physical Therapy: JAPTA,* Vol. 49, No. 5 (May 1969), 470-475.
3. McGarey, William A., *Edgar Cayce and the Palma Christi,* Virginia Beach, Va., A.R.E Press, 1970.
4. Reilly, Harold J., "Drugless Therapy from the Edgar Cayce Records," *The Searchlight,* Vol. 12, No. 6 (June 1960).
5. Reilly, Harold J., "Healing Begins in the Mind," *The Searchlight,* Vol. 12, No. 2 (February 1960).
6. Reilly, Harold J., "The Physical Body Is the Result," *The Searchlight,* Vol. 6, No. 9 (July 1954).

7. Turner, Gladys Davis, "Osteopathy from the Edgar Cayce Records," *The Searchlight,* Vol. 2, No. 12 (December, 1959).
8. Turner, Gladys Davis, "The Power of Attitudes in Serious Diseases," *The Searchlight,* Vol. 11, No. 8 (August 1959).
9. Turner, Gladys Davis, "The Power of Attitudes in Serious Diseases: Part 2—Arthritis," *The Searchlight,* Vol. 12, No. 11 (November 1960.)
10. Wakim, Khalil G., "Physiologic Effects of Massage" in *Massage, Manipulation & Traction,* Sidney Licht, ed., New Haven, Conn., Elizabeth Licht, 1960.

Teething
Ipsab has lots of uses (see "Ipsab—An Herbal Remedy for Gum Problems"), but Mayo Hotten, D.O., tells us of a "new" one. One of his patients started his granddaughter on Ipsab rubs, with a Q-tip, for troubles in teething. It was highly successful, taking away the pain and irritation. Apparently, it also helped the parents to sleep at night!

Childbirth and Castor Oil
One of our correspondents, who has been an active A.R.E. member for many years, wrote about his experience with castor oil packs as an adjunct to childbirth. He reports that his wife "used the castor oil packs during labor with our second child, and she very strongly feels that it was responsible for the brief delivery—four hours as opposed to 27 hours labor with our first child. Furthermore, we have given the newborn castor oil rubs daily and find her to be a most remarkable baby in her disposition and also very alert."

Canker Sores in the Mouth
These seem to respond well to local applications of Atomidine, followed by Glyco-Thymoline. Dr. Harvey Rose reported on his enlarging file of such cases at the A.R.E. Medical Symposium. Our business manager benefited from the information and found that the lesion on his tongue cleared up within three days.

EXERCISES FOR TODAY

In our present-day society with its emphasis on mental achievement and physical ease, it is difficult for the individual to keep his body in good shape. Some rather special complaints now affect large numbers of people. The following excerpts from the Edgar Cayce readings have been chosen with the idea that they may be of help to those suffering from these conditions. For others, these exercises could be the means of forestalling such complaints.

As most individuals find, the business of keeping well and physically fit is something to be worked at . . .
First, then, take those precautions as respecting same. Take time to rest, to exercise, to keep in a physically fit condition.
849-18

. . . to overexercise any portion not in direct need of same, to the detriment of another, is to hinder rather than to assist through exercise. Exercise is wonderful, and necessary—and little or few take as much as is needed, in a systematic manner. Use common sense. Use discretion.
283-1

. . . a regular setting up exercise will build muscles. You'd better first fix the body, however, before you undertake any systematic setting up exercise. When begun, it should be adhered to consistently . . .
4008-1

Morning and evening

Of morning upon arising take the head and neck exercise; circulating the head first, very slowly, three to five times to the right, then three to five times to the left. Sitting or standing erect, bend the head *backward* slowly, just as far as it can, three times; then forward three times; then to the left three times; then to the right three times. Take the *time* to do these, slowly but definitely; not as rote but as doing an act for the accomplishing of a purpose.

Then the exercise of the arms, as straight out from the body, either side. Then bend backward, with the arms attempting to touch in the back; three, four, five times. Then to the front, or from the back to the front . . .

In the evening just before retiring, take rather the circular motion exercise of the body from the hips *up,* first; standing erect, hands on hip, circling the body as from the hips. Then bend forward, without bending knees, the fingers toward the floor. Then standing erect, hands on hips, take the circular motion again of the head and neck.   1131-3

Of morning, and upon arising especially (and don't sleep too late!)—and before dressing, so that the clothing is loose or the fewer the better—standing erect before an open window, breathe deeply; gradually raising hands *above* the head, and then with the circular motion of the body from the hips bend forward; breathing *in* (and through the nostrils) as the body rises on the toes—breathing very deep; *exhaling suddenly* through the *mouth; not* through the nasal passages. Take these for five to six minutes. Then as these progress, gradually *close* one of the nostrils (even if it's necessary to use the hand— but if it is closed with the left hand, raise the right hand; and when closing the right nostril with the right hand, then raise the left hand) *as* the breathing *in* is accomplished. Rise, and [then perform] the circular motion of the body from the hips, and bending forward; *expelling* as the body reaches the lowest level in the bending towards the floor (expelling through the mouth, suddenly). See?

Then of an evening, just before retiring—with the feet braced against the wall, circle the torso by resting on the hands. Raise and lower the body not merely by the hands but more from the torso, and with more of a circular motion of the pelvic organs to strengthen the muscular forces of the abdomen. Not such an activity as to cause strain, but a gentle, circular motion to the right two to three times, and then to the left.

Take these exercises night and morning; the standing and the bending and circling with the breathing of a morning; the circular motion of the pelvis and the torso of the body with the feet braced, using the hands, of an evening; doing these, of course, with the clothing loose or removed, so that there are the full movements.   1523-2

Constipation

Q-4. Why have I not overcome constipation?
A-4. Not sufficient activity of the system in the lower

portion. *This,* for this body, will overcome it. Not so much other than the diet that's been taken. Of morning—upon arising—exercise the body only from the waist up, of morning—see? Before retiring, the circular motion of the body from the diaphragm down.   69-2

Feet

It would be well if there would be this exercise night and morning; night before retiring . . . and of morning just before putting on the hose . . .

Stand erect (without anything on the feet, of course). Then raise the arms, gently, slowly, over the head—directly over the head. Then gradually rise on the toes. Then, as the body relaxes or lowers itself, lower the hands also—the hands extending in front of the body. Then rock back upon the heels, with the hands extended sufficiently to strain or to exercise the bursa of the heel, or those portions of the heel *and* the arch, you see, to aid in strengthening.   1771-3

Head and neck

For those conditions with the sympathetic system, if the body would take the head and neck exercise, we will find it will relieve those little tensions which have been indicated as part of conditions in head, eyes, mouth and teeth. All of these will respond to regular exercise of body and neck. It doesn't take long, but don't hurry through with it. But do regularly of morning take the time before dressing, rise on the toes slowly and raise the arms easily at the same time directly above the head, pointing straight up. At the same time bend head back just as far as you can. When let down gentle from this you see, we make for giving a better circulation through the whole area from the abdomen, through the diaphragm, through the lungs, head and neck. Then let down, put the head forward just as far as it will come on the chest, then raise again at the top, bend the head to the right as far as it will go down. When rising again, bend the head to the left. Then standing erect, hands on hips, circle the head, roll around to the right two or three times, then straighten self. Again hands off the hip, down gently, rise again, down again, then circle to the opposite side. We will find we will change all of these disturbances through the mouth, head, eyes and the activities of the whole body will be improved. Open your mouth as you go up and down also.
                                                        470-37

Hemorrhoids

Then—each morning and each evening, before there is anything binding about the body of morning and *after* disrobing in the evening—for at least three to five minutes take this exercise: Rise gently on the toes (and this without shoes, of course), and at the same time raise the hands high above the head, then lean forward as much as possible without losing balance. Do this slowly and consistently.   563-5

Posture

Mornings upon arising, take for two minutes an exercise in this manner—where the body, standing with the feet flat on the floor, gently rises to the toes, at the same time bringing the arms high above the head. Then bring these as far back as possible or practical, swinging both arms back. Then gradually bring them towards the front, then let down. Breathe *in* as the body rises, and *out* as the body brings the hands to the front, slowly. Do this three or four times each morning . . . This is an excellent exercise for posture . . . 1773-1

Prostatitis

Dr. Harold J. Reilly is a legend in the story of Edgar Cayce's life and readings, and it is always a pleasure to report on one of his simple remedies—in this instance a very useful one in the case of prostatitis. In a letter to a friend of mine, Dr. Reilly said to strike the buttocks with doubled-up fists rather sharply about twelve times, three times daily. And, as an additional help: "Lie on a blanket on the floor (not the bed). Bring knees up and lift the buttocks up and down hitting the floor with a little force (not too much at first) in order to create a vibration through the pelvic region, four times daily to start with and then four times twice a day a bit later. Then increase the 'bumps' until you are doing eight bumps twice a day. Take a month to reach the eight by adding one bump per week, see?" That's Reilly, not Cayce.

AN INTRODUCTION TO HERBS IN THE EDGAR CAYCE READINGS

by Cecil Nichols

The science-oriented twentieth century seems to have come the full circle as researchers try to isolate the healing properties of various plants, and look for the truth long preserved in folklore. Richard Lucas's book, *Nature's Medicines,* is a fascinating account of folk remedies and their use to modern medicine. Although the lowly weeds, seeds and herbs may seem to be enjoying recently attained respectability, a glance at the indices to the Edgar Cayce readings indicates that their role was important in the prescriptions that came through the psychic source. Indexed at this time are more than 7,000 references to herbs, and research into this material has just begun. No positive conclusions are possible yet, not only because of the tremendous number of references to be checked, but also because of the varying combinations recommended. Thus far, the writer has not found a reading which prescribed a single herb not combined with others.

In most cases the specific curative action of the herb was not described, so reading 636-1 is unusual. The beauty shop operator for whom the reading was given in 1934 asked:

Q-4. Please give me a formula for a medicine to be taken internally to restore natural color to hair.
A-4. This would necessarily be put up under the direction of a pharmacist, unless it was formed into an organization for the manufacture of same; which would be a combination in these proportions, whether making two ounces or four hundred gallons:
To 4 ounces of Simple Syrup, add:

Lactated Pepsin	**1 ounce**
Black Snake Root Extract	**¼ ounce**

Essence of Wild Ginseng	¼ ounce
Atomidine	40 minims
Extract of Liver (preserved in alcohol, of course, or Armour's Liver Extract)	½ ounce
Grain Alcohol	¼ ounce

The dosage of this would be half a teaspoon three times each day, just after meals, for periods of ten days with five-day rest periods. This taken in such a manner over a period of several months will be effective to glands, to those secretions that will not only make a digestion that will be much improved in health but—with any good scalp treatment, especially such as we have indicated—it'll turn graying hairs back to normal; or where it has been streaked even by various forms of dyes, its *growth* will come normal.

Q-5. Please give me a formula to improve and recondition the nails.

A-5. There is not much better than that already prepared by Cutex for the care of the nails, provided the glands (which are from the thyroids, of course) are producing the proper amount of secretions in the system. So, then, what you use to care for the hair will care for the nails also, you see; for they are the *outgrowth* of the same secretions in the system. While there may be occasions when a person with very thin or brittle nails may have very excellent hair, it's because such persons eat their own nails!   636-1

After finishing the questions, Gertrude Cayce started with the waking suggestion, but Edgar Cayce continued:

To turn again to why such a formula as given would affect the body-functionings, as to change the outward activity of the functioning of glands in a body:

The Syrup, surely, is the carrier.

The Pepsin is active such that the ingredients given may be effective upon the basic influences within the body that would produce in the varied offices of the body those proper functionings to stimulate in the proper proportions the activities of the cuticle and the epidermis.

So the basis of not only the complexions of body would be changed as to be more in a healthful and thus in an activative force to beautifying of that which is to man his crown of strength and to woman her head of beauty; for to man hair in the head is as strength—to women is as beauty.

Then, the Essence of the Black Snake Root is an active principle with the lacteal ducts that make for secretions in the system that stimulate a capillary circulation.

Aided in same and purified through the Wild Ginseng Essence, that is—according to the ancients—the basis of the stimulation of life in its very essence in the body of man.

The Atomidine—that is activative in the glands, especially the thyroid, the adrenal and all the ductless activities through the atomic forces in iodine, the one basic force with potash—makes for a balance throughout the functionings of the body itself.

While the Extract of Liver with the preservatives, in the activities with the other portions of the body, become beautifiers. Hence, proportioned as indicated, are activative with a body—healthy; the nails, the cuticle, the epidermis, and the adorning of the beauty of the body—*beautiful!*

We are through.   636-1

The formula given in A-4 of this reading contains two ingredients which would normally be classified as herbs: Black Snake Root and Ginseng. "... the Essence of the Black Snake Root is an active principle with the lacteal ducts that make for secretions in the system that stimulate a capillary circulation..."

According to Lucas, Snake Root (*Rauwolfia*) is an herb known for its ability to alleviate nervous depression—its roots have been chewed among East Indian and African natives for 30 centuries. The isolation of Reserpine from Snake Root in 1952 resulted in the modern tranquilizer. In olden times this plant was purported to cure snake bite, and no doubt from this source its name sprang.

. . . the Wild Ginseng Essence, that is—according to the ancients—the basis of the stimulation of life in its very essence in the body of man.   636-1

...Ginger and Ginseng...act directly with the organs as are affected by the gland production in system.   1278-1

Stimulation from the Wild Ginseng is to the gastric flow but acts primarily upon the glands of the gastric flow for an activity to the thyroid, to the ducts and glands within the liver area itself as stimulated by the Indian Turnip ...   1019-1

Thus, according to the Edgar Cayce readings, the effect of Ginseng on the human body is to stimulate the glands.

Historically, the Chinese have been using Ginseng for 50 centuries. In fact, the name Ginseng is compounded from two

Chinese words meaning man-plant. The roots somewhat resemble the shape of man, some specimens remarkably so. Lucas reports that the Chinese consider Ginseng as a panacea for all diseases, and assert that the herb overcomes disease by building general vitality and resistance, especially strengthening the endocrine glands. Centuries of experience have convinced these people that Ginseng rejuvenates and restores vitality to glandular organs by feeding them radioactive elements that this herb has been shown to contain. Lucas says that the Russians investigated Ginseng in the pre-World War II years at the Institute of Experimental Medicine of the U.S.S.R. for the purpose of discovering whether the purported remarkable properties of the herb were due to its radioactive content. They learned that a certain variety of wild Ginseng, which flourished in the Sikhote-Alin mountain range, could only be grown in radioactive soil. Soviet investigators showed that the roots contained many radioactive properties, including the ability to emit warmth. The beginning of World War II interrupted these investigations. C.S. Ogolevec's *Cyclopedia Dictionary of Medical Botany* reports that during the Korean War millions of dollars' worth of Korean Ginseng was sent to the U.S.S.R. when the northern armies overran Korea. Subsequent research by the Russians showed that Ginseng strengthens the heart and nervous system and increases the hormones. Which hormones were increased was not stated. Analysis showed Ginseng to contain Panaxin, Panaquilom, Schingenin and other compounds.

The above references certainly appear to substantiate the statements in the readings regarding the effect of Ginseng on the human glandular system. Several varieties of Ginseng are known to medicine. The Wild Manchurian variety, which grows only in the Sikhote-Alin Mountains, is considered the best. The readings seemed to differ from "medical opinion" on the point of which Ginseng is superior. I say "seemed to differ" because the readings researched to date appear to use the terms Ginseng and Wild Ginseng interchangeably and failed to state the particular variety. Several persons who were intimately involved with the readings during the time they were given stated that the Wild American Ginseng (*Panax quinquefolius*) was used. It is almost certain that should this choice have been mistaken, it would have been so stated in subsequent readings. No such references have been uncovered to date. The position of the readings in this respect may be similar to their philosophy regarding the advisability of eating only foods grown in the vicinity where a person resides. The following extract illustrates this point:

> ... use more of the products of the soil that are grown in the immediate vicinity. These are better for the body than any specific set of fruits, vegetables, grasses, or whatnot.
>
> 4047-1

Another example of the usage of herbs appears in this reading, given on October 28, 1929, for an adult female suffering from general debilitation.

We would prepare, then, this:
To ½ gallon of rain water, or distilled water, we would add:

Wild Cherry Bark	2 ounces
Sarsaparilla Root	1 ounce
Wild Ginger	1 dram
Ginseng	1 dram
Cinchona Bark	½ ounce
(That's Quinine Bark—Cinchona, see?)	
Buchu Leaves	1 dram
Elder Flower	1 ounce

Reduce this by simmering, or slow boiling, to ½ the quantity. Strain while still warm. Best were this strained through the filter paper. Then add, 2 ounces of grain alcohol, with 2 drams Balsam of Tolu cut in same.

Shake solution together before the dose is taken. The dose should be [a] teaspoonful 3 times each day, taken preferably half an hour *after* the meals—and eat the meals; but be mindful of the *character* of the meals. There should *not* be any white bread. There may be whole wheat or rye, or even the mixtures of same. There should be the *juices,* or soups of the vegetables, in which all of the protein from the meats should be put; but not much of the meats, if any. These, though, may be taken at *times,* when the body feels it absolutely necessary . . .

Q-4. *What causes backaches, and what can be done to help?*

A-4. With the application of the properties as given, we will find the changes—for these are the effects of the various properties, and—as will be seen—these have been given due consideration. The effect of this combination in the system is: In that, first, of the barks, to *clarify* the blood as related to the respiratory system, or that through the activity of the lungs, in the carbon condition created in system. In those of the Ginger and Ginseng, act directly with the organs as are affected by the gland production in system. Those of the Quinine Bark, are those that are to *clarify* the blood supply, as is related to the liver. That of the Buchu leaves and Elder flower, are for those effects in the kidneys and the pelvic organs. Those others are the *carriers* and *assimilating* forces in the system. See?

1278-1

"... the barks ... *clarify* the blood as related to the respiratory system ..." The barks referred to are the Wild Cherry and the Cinchona.

Lucas reports that all parts of the Wild Cherry tree have been used as folk medicine and that in some countries a tea made from the bark was employed as an astringent. He does not mention quinine.

"That of the Buchu leaves and Elder flower, are for those effects in the kidneys and the pelvic organs." Buchu leaves are from certain plants of the genera *Barosma* and *Diosma* and are commonly used as a diuretic and diaphoretic. Lucas reports that the Indians made a tea of Elder flowers as a colic remedy, and that folk medicine employed Elder tea as a diuretic.

... there is within the grasp of man all that in nature that is ... an antidote for *every* poison, for every ill in the individual experience, if there will but be applied nature, natural sources.

2396-2

Witch Hazel as Therapy

A few months ago, I heard from a correspondent of mine in Detroit who had been afflicted with a dermatitis of the palm of her hand for some twelve years. After reading Jess Stearn's book, *Edgar Cayce, the Sleeping Prophet,* she decided to use witch hazel on it in the manner described therein. She reported "great improvement" with just two weeks of this treatment. *Hamamelis virginiana* is a small shrub, the leaves and bark of which are used to make witch hazel. There are two forms of the medication, alcoholic and nonalcoholic. Witch hazel has been used internally for dysentery, but is most often used as an astringent or as a wash for burns, bruises, skin irritations and other forms of external inflammation. It has also been used for sore mouths and inflamed eyes. We repeat—simple things are often the best!

BLESSED RAGWEED—
The Most Hated of Weeds

by Robert O. Clapp

The thought of ripening ragweed makes millions uncomfortable—people whose noses run and eyes water during the pollen-bearing months. They know that with the beginning of the fall season they have many days and nights of discomfort ahead of them. In reading 644-1 Cayce refers to ragweed as "the most hated of the weeds"—and rightly so to those who suffer from hay fever. Although many people have a loathing for this weed, and even though the herb books rarely ever mention ragweed, the Cayce readings did not neglect it. There are over 125 references to ragweed in the readings indexed under *Prescriptions: Ragweed*.

Scanning the index cards we find ragweed referred to in connection with many diseases and ailments: catarrh, diabetes, digestion, epilepsy, intestinal problems, nephritis, pelvic disorders, psoriasis, rheumatism, etc. It is a specific for appendicitis. But the vast majority of references to ragweed are in connection with an incoordination between assimilations and eliminations. Basically, then, the herb has to do with the stimulation of the eliminative process.

In 953-18 Cayce said, "[Take] small quantities of [ragweed], occasionally, to assist in the proper assimilation . . ." and in 903-35 he said, "[ragweed] is one of the best eliminants with a vegetable base. But it must be chosen very young, and the leaves alone chewed—but don't spit it out because it is bitter! It's not poisonous, and it is a good eliminant . . ."

Mrs. [454] was told that her physical condition was very good in most respects but warned that there was a tendency for the body "to overtax self" which might lead to diabetes. Continuing, her reading said:

[If there will] be taken in the system, at regular intervals, those properties that are not habit forming, neither are they

45

effective towards creating the condition where cathartics are necessary for the activities through the alimentary canal—whether related to the colon or the jejunum, or ileum—yet these will change the vibrations in such a manner as to keep clarified the assimilations, and aid the pancreas, the spleen, the liver and the hepatic circulation, in keeping a normal equilibrium. These properties would be found in those of the ambrosia weed, made in this manner:

To 6 ounces of distilled water, add 3 ounces of the *green* ragweed, or ambrosia weed. Steep for sufficient period to reduce this to half the quantity. Then strain, adding to this 2 ounces of simple syrup, with 1 ounce of grain alcohol. Shake the solution before the dose is taken. The dose would be half a teaspoonful twice each day, when the period for taking has arisen—or take it about once each month, for three or four days. This will aid the digestive system, will aid the whole of the *eliminating* system.   454-1

A number of factors work in favor of ragweed: It is plentiful and cheap, within the grasp of anyone. You can gather it yourself or buy it dried from an herbal supply house. It is not poisonous or harmful or, according to Cayce, habit forming. Making the above formula is easy. Distilled water may be purchased at any drugstore. A simple syrup is made with equal parts of sugar and water; the preservative, grain alcohol, can be purchased at any liquor store.

One of the curious things about plant classification is the names given to certain herbs. *Cascara sagrada* is otherwise known as sacred bark; a synonym for the castor oil plant is the *Palma Christi*—the hand of Christ; *Buchu leaves* are otherwise called *Diosma,* meaning divine order. (Incidentally, all of these plants figure prominently as prescription items in the Cayce readings.) In Greek mythology ambrosia was the food of the gods, and some translators interpret ambrosia as "not mortal." Is it coincidence, then, that the generic name for the lowly ragweed is *ambrosia,* a word used interchangeably with ragweed in the readings? Could it be that the ancients knew of an intrinsic value in ragweed that modern man who wages chemical warfare with the plant hasn't yet discovered?

A variation of the eliminative formula, indexed also under *Incoordination of Assimilations and Eliminations* appears in this excerpt:

To meet the needs of the conditions at the present, we would first cleanse the system with a mild cathartic; preferably that as would be found in combining the ragweed with senna. This combination: To 3 ounces of ragweed add 8 ounces distilled or rain water. Reduce to half the quantity. Strain, adding sufficient alcohol to preserve same. Adding *then* to same 2 grains of senna. Shaking well together, the dose would be [a] teaspoonful every evening until at least half to two-thirds of the quantity is taken.   3826-1

Here a more sophisticated formula was recommended:

In 4 ounces of simple syrup we would add:
Tincture of Ambrosia Weed	2 ounces
Tincture of Stillingia	¼ ounce
Tincture of Wild Ginseng	¼ ounce
Syrup of Sarsaparilla Compound	½ ounce

Shake the solution together before the dosage is taken. The dose would be half a teaspoonful three times each day. The addition of these properties in the system will change the digestive forces as to assimilation, causing or producing less of an acid in the digestive system, clarifying a coordinating force (that is, with the correction and the vibration added with same) between the liver and the kidneys, and making for a nearer normal balance.   666-1

To say that modern man has neglected ragweed is not entirely accurate. There are perhaps fifty to one hundred references to Simmons' Liver Regulator in the index to the readings—an item no longer on the market—and Simmons' had as its basic ingredient ragweed along with licorice and cascara sagrada. A fifty-two-year-old woman, bothered by sciatica tendencies, asked:

Q-3. Have the sweats and massages been given correctly?
A-3. They have been given very well, but not in just the manner indicated.
We would keep up the eliminations. The liver needs stirring more, see? These we would carry through to stir the liver to better activity; not with the minerals as much as with vegetables. As we find, the Simmons' Liver Regulator now would be the better, whether it is in the powder or in the liquid form. But these we would keep up, so that there are at least two or three eliminations daily.
Q-4. Did the colonic do any good (apparently it only irritated)?
A-4. It did good. Thus the needs for the colon to be drained so as to allow the better assimilations for the body.

Q-5. Is the mineral oil I am taking good for me?

A-5. Not unless the rest of the pockets of the colon are cleansed.

Q-6. Should I take olive oil, say a teaspoonful with each meal?

A-6. This is very well, but what is needed is to cleanse the colon and the secretions of the liver and the gall duct increased. Thus the form of vegetable forces indicated. For this is ambrosia weed, with sufficient of the licorice and cascara to aid in stimulating and in fitting it for the body—though the better way would be to eat the ragweed itself!

404-13

Another reference to Simmons' follows:

Then, after the [castor oil] packs have been given for five days, begin with taking small doses of the essence of ambrosia weed. *Preferably* this would be taken green, or *new;* prepared in this manner:

Put about half an ounce of the green ambrosia weed in a pint of water. Let this come thoroughly to a boil (after the weed has been bruised and put in the water, you see). Then take off and strain; and to the quantity that is left—which would be about two-thirds of a pint, you see—add one ounce of pure grain alcohol, that it may be preserved.

The dose of this would be half a teaspoonful three times each day (after the meals), until there are *thorough* eliminations through the alimentary canal from the taking of same; that it may act upon the liver.

This is better for the body than taking even the Simmons' Liver Regulator; which is of the same, but is combined with licorice and other compounds that, for *this* body, would *not* be so well.

1880-1

One can conjecture that Cayce saw the day when Simmons' Liver Regulator would no longer be available. In a reading for a seventy-six-year-old man suffering from pneumonia, Cayce again gave an alternative which can easily be compounded.

The Calcidin is well, as is also the Alophen, but *better still* would it be were those properties for the *eliminant* be oils—*with* those of either the ragweed or the Simmons' Liver Regulator, which is ragweed and licorice and a little senna. These would be *more* effective, and the *oil necessary* to take the inflammation out, or through the intestinal tract...

Q-2. How much oil should be given?

A-2. Two teaspoonsful of the Russian White Oil and *half* a teaspoonful—in about half an hour afterwards—of the Simmons' Liver Regulator, or it may be compounded in that of the ragweed, or ragweed tea, made in *this* manner: This would be preferable to make it from the original.

To 6 ounces of distilled water, add ambrosia weed 2½ ounces. Steep, or slow boil, for 20 minutes. Strain off. Then add:

Licorice in solution	½ ounce
Syrup of Sarsaparilla Compound	¼ ounce

Cut ½ dram Balsam of Tolu in 2 ounces of alcohol and add to same.

The dose then would be, after the oil, see—about half to three-quarters of an hour—half a teaspoonful. Take until there is a thorough evacuation from the bowel.   304-18

Anyone who has ever tasted ragweed will know that it is bitter as gall, which probably explains why licorice or syrup were included in various formulas. Those who like to take shortcuts and avoid the bother of collecting the necessary ingredients, the measuring, straining, mixing, etc., might simply bend over and pluck a tender tip of ragweed, chew and swallow.

It wouldn't be fair to discuss ragweed without including something for the hay fever sufferers. Reading for such an individual, Mr. Cayce told him how he could build up a natural resistance to ragweed during July and August so that by September there would be bettered conditions for the body.

Now, as we find, there are conditions which tend to disturb the body at specific periods. Hence, as is indicated, there are certain seasons or periods when the vibrations of the body, or the relationships which are established in the nerve centers, are such as to cause the body to become allergic to conditions which exist in or under certain environs, or certain pressure experienced by climatic reactions in the body.

These reactions come from what may be called or set up as vibrations in certain centers between sympathetic and cerebrospinal system, and thus the body in such periods is subject to conditions which manifest in irritation to mucous membranes of the nasal passage and throat, bronchi and larynx, or, as sometimes called, rose fever or such natures. These, for this body, are particularly from the ragweed.

Thus, we would find in this particular season, before there is the blossoming of same, the body should take quantities of this weed. Brew same, prepare, take internally and thus war or ward against the activity of this upon the body itself.

Then, through the period, also take that as an antiseptic reaction upon the nerves of the nasal passages, or the olfactory nerves of the body.

These will prevent, then, the recurrent conditions which have been and are a part of the experience of the body. This will enable the body to become immune because of the very action of this weed upon the digestive system, and the manner it will act with the assimilating body, too. Well, just don't get too heavy, for it will make for an increase in the amount of assimilation and distribution of food values for the body.

Thus we would prepare the compound in this manner: Take a pint cup, gather the tender leaves of the weed, don't cram in but just fill level. Put this in an enamel or a glass container and then the same amount (after cleansing, of course, don't put dirt and all in but put in same amount by measure) of distilled water, see? Reduce this to half the quantity by very slow boiling, not hard but slow boiling, strain and add sufficient grain alcohol as a preservative.

Begin and take it through the fifteen days of July and the whole of August, daily, half a teaspoonful each day.

Thus, we will find better eliminations, we will find better assimilation, we will find better distribution of the activities of foods in the body.

Then, use through the latter portion of August and September, this as a combination: Prepare in the manner indicated, putting together the ingredients only in the order named. First we would prepare a bottle with a large mouth, two vents through the cork and these vents capable of being corked themselves with a small cork. Neither of the vents is to enter the solution, so use a six-ounce container. In this container put four ounces of grain alcohol (at least 90% proof), then add in the order named:

Oil of Eucalyptus	20 minims
Rectified Oil of Turp	5 minims
Compound Tincture of Benzoin	15 minims
Oil of Pine Needles	10 minims
Tolu in Solution	10 minims

When this is to be used, shake the solution together, remove the corks from the vent, inhale deep through the nostril so as to enter the nasal passages, also to the upper and back portions of throat, both passages. Shake between each deep inhalation.

Do these and we'll have better conditions for the body. Do for the body-forces use wheat germ in the morning meal with the cereal, which may be taken a teaspoonful over a good bowl of cereal, then add the cream and a little sugar if desired.

Do these and we'll have bettered conditions for this body, [5347].

Ready for questions.

Q-1. To the amount of the ragweed we would use how much alcohol?

A-1. That should be done by the prescriptionist or the chemist, just to preserve same.   5347-1

As we study our surroundings it becomes evident that nothing in nature is intrinsically bad, it is the way we use a substance that determines its value. We see this concept so often supported in the Cayce readings: red wine is a blood builder; cobra venom a medicine; the deadly foxglove (digitalis) and castor beans are a heart remedy in the first instance and a varied healer in the second. The same is true of ragweed. Rightly understood, it can be of great value to mankind. Aside from its healing powers the significance of ragweed in the readings might well be to emphasize our need to understand how objects in nature can be used constructively in the spirit of "subdue the earth and replenish it." If we can come to understand, through application, the helpful use of weeds, our encounter with ragweed can indeed be a blessing.

Castor Oil vs. Drugs

The use of castor oil in treating drug overdose is perhaps the latest therapeutic triumph registered by the plant, which the imaginative people of the Middle Ages called the Palma Christi. It has been reported from Canada (by Dr. Michael Diamond) and from the University of Medicine in Miami, Florida, that individuals who have attempted suicide by taking large overdoses of drugs are being given quantities of castor oil greatly exceeding the ounce or two usually taken as a cathartic or for inducing labor in pregnant women. Nearly a pint is administered twice a day, and patients who were comatose and expected to remain so for four or five days recovered in 24 hours. Some physicians believe that the castor oil absorbs the drugs, quickly removing them from the system. Thus the harmful effects of the body's prolonged exposure to drugs are prevented. Some doctors add charcoal tablets to the castor oil; this acts as a detoxifying agent and enhances the curative effect. This treatment could well save the lives of many who have taken large drug overdoses.

THE HEALING POWERS OF SAFFRON TEA

by Robert O. Clapp

If one were to use as a guide the number of times an item is mentioned in the Edgar Cayce readings, it would be safe to say that every avid devotee of the readings should drink saffron tea! Of the 250 times the herb saffron is called for, approximately 200 refer to its use as a tea—more than any other tea mentioned in the readings—ranking fifth among the herbs named. Teas which appear often in the readings are watermelon seed, mullein, camomile and ragweed in that order, but saffron leads the list by a wide margin.

Knowing why saffron was recommended, for what ailments and for what purposes, leads us to conclude that it can be useful to many of us. Were one interested in specific health advice, the place to look would be complete readings on a particular malady (psoriasis or diabetes, for instance) or collections of readings (*Circulating Files*) rather than extracts taken out of context. For our purposes here, though, we will consider broadly the part saffron plays as a healing agent and not necessarily the complete regimen to be followed in curing specific ailments. That is to say, these extracts should stimulate a concerned person to look further.

One of the remarkable aspects of the readings is the way the Cayce source prescribes an herb or an herbal remedy and then goes on to explain in detail what the item does to bring about healing.

The activity of this [saffron tea] upon the gastric flow of the stomach and duodenum and through the alimentary canal will tend to allay, and to work with the activities that supply the mucous membrane flow along the canal itself, thus aiding the body. [Psoriasis] 3112-1

Also during the period when the colonic irrigations and the

osteopathic treatments are being given, we would take a great deal of the saffron tea (made from American saffron), that it may aid in creating better activity through the peristaltic movement of the eliminating system. [Poor Eliminations]

1930-1

And about twice a day (this between the meals) have half an ounce of yellow saffron tea; not too strong. This as we find will prevent the accumulations of gas and the inflammation to be absorbed by the activities of these properties through the system. [Intestines: Gas]

428-11

The saffron tea is very well as an intestinal antiseptic . . . [Measles]

487-26

The extracts quoted above enlarge on *why* saffron was recommended—"creating better activity through the peristaltic movement of the eliminating system," "prevent the accumulations of gas and the inflammation to be absorbed," "an intestinal antiseptic"—rather than just because the tea was recommended in connection with a particular ailment.

The major topics under which saffron tea is indexed are psoriasis (14 references), lacerations (19), eliminations (13), assimilations and eliminations: incoordination (14), toxemia (14) and ulcers (21). From this list we can see that saffron works on the stomach and intestines and is an aid to those skin ailments the cause of which is a malfunction in the alimentary canal.

What is this marvelous herb and how readily available is it? The readings were not specific, but apprently the herb referred to was *Carthamus tinctorius,* which is also known as saffron, bastard saffron, safflower and American saffron. The other saffron, the true saffron, is *Crocus sativus.* It is grown in western Asia, Spain, France and Austria. When compacted it is also called hay saffron.

Of *Carthamus tinctorius* Myers tells us it "is cultivated in England and America and the countries surrounding the Mediterranean Sea. The orange-red florets are the official parts."[1] Culbreath indicates that *Carthamus tinctorius* is cultivated in India and America.[2] Kloss, likewise, refers to *Carthamus tinctorius* as American saffron, false saffron, bastard saffron, and safflower, but does not mention *Crocus sativus* at all.[3] Harris calls *Carthamus tinctorius* American or Dyer's Saffron and says that it is often substituted for the expensive saffron (by which we assume he means *Crocus sativus*), which he calls true or Spanish saffron.[4] Another distinction made by Culpepper is meadow saffron or *Colchicum autumnale,* but in describing saffron (*Crocus sativus*) he says, "it grows in various parts of the world but it is no better than that which grows in England."[5]

Probably the definitive treatise on herbs is *A Modern Herbal,* Vols. I and II by Mrs. M. Grieve.[6] In describing safflower, *Carthamus tinctorius,* she says, "This plant is not in any way related to saffron, though the flowers are used similarly. (It largely replaces the use of saffron owing to the large price of the latter.) . . . Another common use of safflower is in adulterating saffron." Like saffron, Mrs. Grieve says, *Carthamus tinctorius* is used in children's and infants' complaints—measles, fevers and skin disorders. The best saffron comes from Spain. Approximately 4,320 flowers are required for an ounce and medicinally it is carminative (aids in expelling gas), diaporetic (promotes perspiration), and emmenagogue (stimulates menstruation).

It may be that the two herbs, *Carthamus tinctorius* and *Crocus sativus,* are interchangeable, but on the basis of what we can glean from the readings *Carthamus tinctorius* appears to be what is recommended.

Regarding whether Spanish, Mexican or American saffron is the best, the Cayce source responded: "The American saffron will be found to be most helpful. This is really preferable to the Spanish saffron which is much more expensive." (428-12)

An ounce box of saffron (*Carthamus tinctorius*) used regularly should last a couple of months and is as inexpensive as drinking coffee. As for manner of preparation this extract is typical:

Hence, we would begin taking internally once each day, preferably just before retiring, a cup of saffron tea. Put a pinch of the American saffron in a cup of boiling water, or put it in the cup and pour boiling water over it and allow to stand for thirty minutes (covered during that period, of course). Then strain, cool, and drink. Use a good pinch of saffron, you see, between the thumb and the forefinger, to the cup of boiling water. Make this fresh each time. 3112-1

Psoriasis
Probably the strongest endorsement for saffron is to be found in the psoriasis readings. It is often used in conjunction with

elm water. In his first reading, Mr. [289] asked about this ailment:

Q-4. Please give me the cause and cure for the so-called psoriasis with which I am troubled.

A-4. The cause is the thinning of the walls of the intestinal system, which allows the escaping of poisons—or the absorption of same by the mucous membranes which surround same, and becomes effective in the irritation through the lymph and emunctory reactions in the body.

An effective cure for same is first being mindful of the diet, during the periods when these necessary elements would be given for creating those activities within the system to close such conditions:

In the system we would use elm water and saffron water. These would be taken in the ordinary drinking water, during periods of one, two to three weeks at a time. All the drinking water carrying, then, either a small quantity of elm or the saffron.

For this adds to the assimilating system those properties that become effective to the aiding of building within the system itself those conditions that will overcome such activities in the system.   289-1

Repeating the reference to the thinned conditions of the intestinal system, reading 641-7 (for psoriasis) adds a third remedy often found with saffron and elm—camomile tea.

We would keep to the taking, more often, the saffron tea as indicated; and we would change or alternate this at times with camomile tea. For these tend to form, in the regular activities of the body, the best in the gastric flows for the intestinal disorder.   641-7

Both the saffron and the camomile assist the gastric flow and aid digestion, as stated in other readings.

Miss [2884] was 10 years old when she received her first readings; she was afflicted with abrasions and poor blood coagulation. In the next two years she had two more readings. Although psoriasis wasn't mentioned in the course of the readings, the symptoms were:

These conditions, as we find, exist:

There has for so long a time remained that condition wherein the mucous membranes of the digestive system, and of the intestinal tract even proper—or the walls, are thinned by this impoverishment. Hence a tendency for the lymph and the mucous membranes to pick up, through these small orifices—and through the improper eliminations of the poisons, and create in the lymph and emunctory circulation those as of the rash, or abrasions, as occur on portions of the system; the body attempting to eliminate poisons, yet when the body is impoverished, so that these would not occur, the whole general system suffers under same, and—as the condition is seen—the system has just been a little too much overloaded, so that the digestive and assimilating juices, or assimilating system, are not able to take care of the conditions in a *normal* way and manner. 2884-3

A portion of the treatment included the following:

We would also prepare to be taken of mornings, that of yellow saffron tea. This should be steeped, not too strong, but about a teaspoonful to the pint of water and allowed to brew or steep as tea—see? This may be kept or set aside, strained and set aside in a cool place, and should last for 2 to 3 days, taking a tablespoon of same in a glass, or half a glass, of water—of mornings, see? after the cereal or fruit has been taken.

We also will find that occasionally camomile tea, made in the same way and manner—this used instead of the saffron, will enable the system—with these being kept in the line as has been outlined—to create more of a mucous membrane in the stomach and intestinal system, see? and keep up those rubs as given for the limbs, and we will find changes coming about, betterments for the body. 2884-3

In 745-1 there is again the reference to the healing of the skin being brought about by dealing with the source of the distress, the intestinal tract. This time the yellow saffron and the elm bark are taken in conjunction with olive oil, which is highly recommended as food for the intestines in many other readings.

There are other factors, such as diet, spinal manipulation, and the improvement of the eliminating system, that assist in controlling and overcoming psoriasis. The *Circulating File,* with its excellent commentary by an M.D., should be consulted for the complete treatment.

After mentioning diet in 840-1, Cayce again affirms the efficacy of saffron and elm bark, adds lithia in this case, and summarizes the reaction of all three:

To the normal water that may be had in the surroundings, we

would add to each gallon (to be kept for drinking water, you see) a five-grain lithia tablet. Dissolve this and it would make about the proper proportion, and it would be added and dissolved in same preferably after the ordinary water had been boiled—or had come to a boil and strained or filtered off before used. Then when this is to be taken, once or twice a day we would have just a pinch of the elm bark (between the thumb and forefinger) in a glass of water—the ground elm bark. If it is more preferable, it may be used with a small piece of ice in same; this would be all the better, but stir same and let it stand for a minute or two before it is taken. We would also, from the same type of water, have the yellow saffron—the American saffron is correct, or may be used if so desired. This would be the proportions of about a heaping teaspoonful to a gallon of water. This preferably we would make in an enamel container or in a glass container, preferable to the aluminum. This would be allowed to steep as would tea. Then it may be drawn off and kept as a portion of the drinking water to be taken at the regular intervals when the body desires water. Not that there would never be any of the regular routine or drinking of water outside, but let the most—and as much as possible all—that is taken either carry one or the other of those properties as indicated. This would be the first precaution, for—while it is, of course, slow acting—it will make for a cleansing of the kidneys, a better activity through the alimentary canal, clear those tendencies for the poisons to accumulate through the lymph and emunctory circulation, and overcome these tendencies for toxic forces to arise in the body that affects the body throughout.   840-1

Lacerations

Lacerations are another problem for which saffron tea was part of the healing regimen. Mr. [270]'s condition was diagnosed by his doctor as an ulcer of the duodenal area and on the underside of the stomach. Asked if the diagnosis were correct, the Cayce source replied:

No. These, as we find, have been lacerations and the better the condition will be if there is the following of these suggestions that have been made, making more milk in the diet where it is practical. Keep away from fats and oils, and it will be better. Do use occasionally the charcoal tablets prepared by Kellogg's. These are the better absorbents and will protect the area. Use the saffron tea also . . . once a day, preferably in the evening when ready to retire. This will be well for the condition.   270-49

As is the case with psoriasis, the treatment for stomach lacerations often calls for both elm in water, saffron tea and the intake of olive oil. The series of readings for [348] calls for this combination repeatedly, with several glasses of saffron tea every few days. For [602] the prescription was saffron tea two to three times a day—a good big swallow or a jigger of the solution each time. The strength of the tea was one teaspoonful to a pint of water. Also called for is olive oil two to three times a day in doses of one quarter of a teaspoonful. Another variation given for [667], likewise suffering from stomach lacerations, was two to four glasses of saffron tea per day for five to six days at a time, then leave off three to four days and begin again, the pattern to be repeated for four to five weeks. For his lacerated stomach Mr. [1481] was told to avoid highly seasoned food and alcohol (with the exception of red wine and brown bread in the afternoon). He was to:

Take mornings and evenings *small* quantities—half to a teaspoonful—of pure olive oil.

In the mid-morning and before the afternoon drink (of the red wine), take a teaspoonful of yellow saffron tea. Use the American saffron and brew it just as tea. These properties act upon the gastric flow of the digestive forces, not only with the salivary glands (in the mouth) but the upper portion or cardiac portion of the stomach itself. This mixing with the gastric flow (that is started by the activity of the olive oil—not at the same period, but taken as has been indicated) will reduce the acidity, will prevent or allay the plethora or swelling as produced in the pylorus and through the duodenum; and thus aid the body in better assimilations. 1481-1

Eliminations

Miss [852]'s father wired "Please give reading . . . having trouble with stomach and digestive tract . . ." The reading stated:

As we find, there are some acute conditions arising from a cold and congestion in the liver and in the digestive system itself; with acute conditions through the lower portion of duodenum and the gall duct area; with pains—by lack of digestion—through the alimentary canal.

First, we would apply the castor oil packs. Before these are begun, however—about three hours before—take a good dose of yellow saffron tea, about two and one-half ounces. Put about two pinches of the yellow saffron in a crock and pour the

boiling water over same, allowing it to stand for about ten minutes. Strain and drink. This may be cooled, of course, to make it more palatable.

Then in about three hours after taking the saffron tea, apply the castor oil pack for about an hour. The next day apply again, and then the next.

Then take at least half a teacup of olive oil.   852-18

In this case the saffron was paired with both the olive oil and the castor oil packs.

In a case of overstimulating of kidneys and congestion in the intestinal tract, sage was given along with saffron.

To meet the needs of these would be to set up proper eliminations. Well that the body rest for two to three days, and well that sweats be taken to start capillary eliminations. Taking internally sage and saffron tea, hot—hot as can be taken—and sweat this *through* the body, see? These may be made in the ordinary way and manner as any tea—saffron and sage—and may be taken separate or together, but at least half a pint of each would be taken each day, and a sweat taken, see? *These* will set up elimination, and these will start *proper* eliminations through the alimentary canal.   2597-1

Later Mr. [257] reported, ". . . your tea fixed him [2597] up and the diagnosis was as perfect as could be."

Mrs. [3287] acquired a strep infection after the birth of her child. The infection localized in the kneecap, which left it stiff. She had two operations but in neither case did the knee become moveable. The last doctor she consulted advised her to leave the knee alone, adding that it was better as is than it might be.

Cayce confirmed the strep infection in blood supply. Saffron and mullein tea were prescribed, along with other corrective measures.

Then begin taking (not before) the saffron tea, a cupful each day—or at least two ounces. Put a pinch of the American saffron in a teacup and pour boiling water over it—allow to stand for twenty to thirty minutes—strain and drink. A pinch between the thumb and forefinger, in the cup of boiling water. Drink two ounces of this, once each day.

Also at the same time begin taking mullein tea, prepared in the same manner—one dram to a cup of boiling water, allowed to steep—drinking only an ounce of this, once each day.

                3287-1

In answers to subsequent questions Mrs. [3287] was advised twice that her problem lay in "Poisons in the system as has been indicated that must be eliminated by increasing the eliminations." (3287-2) The saffron tea was a contributing factor in eliminating these poisons.

Afflicted with epilepsy, 11-year-old [4798] was told that there was a need for eliminations to be kept above normal.

These we would keep active with a mild form of stimuli to the respiratory system, especially from the digestive and lymph area, as a mild form of camomile tea, or saffron tea, that is palliative to the digestive system, and that will make for the proper eliminations, preventing the accumulations of drosses that would affect the system in any way by not being eliminated; keeping the intestinal tract rather active, keeping the body quiet, and the diet rather that of the liquid diet. Plenty of the juices of fruits; little or no nuts. Soups or mild broths, with little vegetable—no meats. 4798-1

Assimilations and Eliminations: Incoordination

Advised about stomach pains and rectal bleeding, Mr. [257] in one reading asked:

Q-3. How long should saffron tea be taken, and what does it do for body?

The reply was:

A-3. This should be kept up not in a haphazard manner, but until there is a better condition physically created throughout the alimentary canal. Take it for two, three, four, five days, a week, ten days—leave it off a few days, and then have it prepared again and take again. This is the best manner.

It stimulates better strength through the activities of the lymph and emunctory circulation in the alimentary canal.

Q-4. How long take elm bark, and what does it do for body?

A-4. As indicated, this would be taken when it desires water—or if it sours in the stomach—or because of foods, or those conditions that arise from a condition in the system— leave off.

This again is to supply that coating along the walls of the intestines themselves, as to prevent the strains from which blood has appeared. 257-215

Mr. [556] anticipated a popular question when he asked:

Q-2. *How may he prevent food causing gas?*

A-2. These as just indicated. The specific activity as we find of the saffron as it will work with the gastric activity, especially of the duodenum from which source most of the gas emanates.

Do those.

Then don't eat too fast, and be careful that there are not the combinations where excess quantities of acid-producing or starchy foods are taken. **556-16**

Summary

In concluding we might observe that tea drinking need not be just a social habit. The right tea—or right combination—can be the means of inducing healing. Because the readings were rather specific in telling us what saffron tea does for the body, it should be given consideration as a means of bringing balance to the stomach and intestines when they are not functioning properly. No rare herb, saffron is within the means of almost everyone and easily available. Our slogan might well be, "Take herb tea and see the result!"

FOOTNOTES

[1] Joseph E. Myers, *The Herbalist.* Hackensack, N.J.: Wehman Bros., 1970. (6th printing)

[2] David M.R. Culbreath, *A Manual of Materia Medica and Pharmacology.* Philadelphia: Lea and Febiger, 1927.

[3] Jethro Kloss, *Back to Eden.* New York: Lancer Books, 1971.

[4] Ben Charles Harris, *The Complete Herbal.* Barre, Maine: Barre Publisher, 1972.

[5] *Culpepper's Complete Herbal.* London: W. Foulsham and Co., Ltd.

[6] Mrs. M. Grieve, *A Modern Herbal,* Vols. I & II. New York: Dover Publications, Inc., 1971.

AN ALMOND A DAY
by W.H. Church

I

An updated look at the almond reveals some surprising nutritional facts. These facts, which reflect the latest research findings in the field of human nutrition, are all the more surprising because they focus our attention on the *mineral* constituents in the almond, rather than the more commonly touted vitamin composition (as presently determined). [1]

Although it is not generally realized, the human body can tolerate a vitamin deficiency for a longer period than a deficiency of minerals. While some of these micro-nutrients are only present in the human organism in "trace" amounts, representing an infinitesimal measurement, they often play a crucial role that can have life-or-death consequences. This may help to explain why medical research is now taking a more careful look at the lack or imbalance of certain mineral constituents in our diet. We are becoming increasingly aware that a deficiency of one or more minerals, or an excess of certain others, can be a prime causal factor in cancer and other diseases.

Finally, a review of the current research data now tends to corroborate the unorthodox dietary advice contained in the Edgar Cayce readings about eating one or two almonds a day— or, at most, three—as a cancer preventative:

> . . . and if an almond is taken each day, and kept up, you'll never have accumulations of tumors or such conditions through the body. An almond a day is much more in accord with keeping the doctor away, especially certain types of doctors, than apples.   3180-3

> And know, if ye would take each day, through thy experience, two almonds, ye will never have skin blemishes, ye will never be tempted even in body toward cancer nor

towards those things that make blemishes in the body forces
themselves.   1206-13

... those who would eat two to three almonds each day need
never fear cancer.   1158-31

A skeptic might ask: Why the variation in the number of
almonds recommended? This is easily answered in terms of
"biochemical individuality." It must be remembered that each
of us is unique, not only as to his spiritual and mental makeup
but in the chemistry of his body as well. And since the readings
were given for different individuals, whose biochemical
requirements could differ substantially, what is really
remarkable, perhaps, is that there was not a *wider* variation in
the prescribed number of almonds. Can we reasonably
conclude, therefore, that there is some peculiar potency in the
almond that dictates the need for *no more than two or three
nuts daily?* Would more than that even be undesirable? Could
an excess of almonds actually create a biochemical imbalance
of some kind that, while not necessarily harmful, might
conceivably nullify the beneficial results we are seeking? It's a
provocative concept. Nor is it without precedent in the annals
of nutritional therapy. Yet, it falls more in line with the
outmoded teachings of homeopathy (made popular by Rudolf
Steiner half a century ago) than with the present-day concept of
"mega-doses," which is being pushed with increasing
frequency and has even been adopted by the embattled
practitioners of the controversial Laetrile treatment—a
"vitamin" approach to cancer that has some interesting
similarities to the Cayce almond formula but with one or two
notable differences, as will be discussed later on.
  Before we proceed, let's re-examine that initial quotation
from the readings, contrasting almonds with apples. It may
have a critical bearing on some of our deductions along the
way. As one might suspect, it has an esoteric significance. Here
is the pertinent excerpt in its entirety:

An almond a day is much more in accord with keeping the
doctor away, especially certain types of doctors, than apples.
For the apple was the fall, not the almond—for the almond
blossomed when everything else died. Remember, this is life!
                                                    3180-3

This statement, alluding in a symbolic manner to the relative merits of the almond versus the apple, relies upon a *spiritual* premise to arrive at a material conclusion. Such a mode of deduction is, no doubt, disconcerting to the average scientific mind. Yet it supports a perspective with which the readings were continually concerned. For the readings tell us that spirit and matter are simply different manifestations of the One Force. And every material manifestation in the universe (which must include the almond as well as the apple) has a spiritual counterpart, or archetype, which is the underlying reality. Life, in its essence, is spiritual; and "all healing must come from that within that is of a spiritual import." (1199-2)

At the same time, appropriate *material* applications were commonly recommended in the physical readings, although typically given as an adjunct to advice of a more spiritual nature:

For, all healing comes from the one source. And whether there is the application of foods, exercise, medicine, or even the knife, it is to bring the consciousness of the forces within the body that aid in reproducing themselves—the awareness of Creative or God forces.   2696-1

This means that any dietary recommendations (such as we are concerned with in this article about almonds) were given in the readings primarily to assist the evolving human personality in raising the consciousness in each cell to a recognition of the Divine within. The operative element in the diet might appear at the physical level as a form of nutrient, constituting a vibratory molecular force able to affect the human bioelectric system in such a manner as to raise healing or protective energies within the body forces themselves; at the same time, energies of a higher and more subtle nature, emanating from the activity of the soul forces, must be generated at the mental and spiritual levels in order for a *sustained* sense of wholeness or healing to occur. It was this higher transformation process that was always the underlying aim of any physical therapy recommended by Edgar Cayce in the readings. (Typically, it involves the development of patience, first, and the persistent overcoming of self through active, loving service to others. Daily periods of earnest prayer and meditation are equally important as a means of achieving spiritual growth and gradual integration with the Higher Self.)

More than once, the dietary recommendations found in the readings even included the Cayce apple diet, thus demonstrating the ability of this "condemned" and lowly fruit to attract toxins to itself and thereby rid the human system of unwanted impurities. The symbolic implications of such a diet are certainly intriguing in light of the Genesis story. It is almost as if a kind of "expiation process" might be involved. For, "Remember, all this is life!"; and as each soul-entity finds itself in the developmental phases of a cause-and-effect universe, where it is called upon to meet itself daily, reaping what has been sown, it is provided with the necessary means by a beneficent Creator.

Whatever conclusions we are to draw on the subject, it is interesting to note that outside of their purgative use in the apple diet, the eating of raw apples was definitely not encouraged in the readings.[2] This was apparently because the adsorbent characteristic of the raw apple pulp, when ingested with other foods, causes it to draw off certain useful nutrients from the system along with the toxins.

So much for the apple.

What of the almond and its spiritual significance? To what shall we attribute its unique biodynamic powers, if a single almond a day—or, at most, two or three almonds a day—can function as a cancer preventative and anti-tumor agent? Can certain organic foods (a nut, in this instance) contain a vibratory "life-force" of a special order that is capable of interacting with the human bioelectric system, even as we have already postulated, to stimulate its vibrations? And, finally, do we know why the almond tree and its fruit were once considered sacred, as confirmed in the Old Testament and in the writings of the early Christian Gnostics? These are cogent questions. We will come back to them.

II

In the meantime, let's pause for a less esoteric look at the almond. We can begin with an examination of its recognized nutritional values. (See Table 1.) In a comparison with raw apples, an equal weight of almonds has a surprisingly high level of phosphorus and potassium, in particular, among the mineral factors. But no one is going to eat a cupful of almonds! So we have to compare the nutrients in the apple with those in a single almond—or with two or three almonds, as in Table 2. We can see, for example, that just a couple of almonds supply more phosphorus than a medium-sized apple; goodly amounts of potassium, magnesium and calcium; an appreciable amount of iron; and certain trace minerals—including zinc and copper.

Table 1—A Comparison of Nutritive Values, Almonds vs. Apples*

Constituent	Unit of Meas.	APPLES, RAW 1 med. apple, 150 grams	ALMONDS, DRIED 1 cup, 142 grams (28 nuts per oz.)	SINGLE ALMOND 1½**
Water	%	84.4	4.7	4.7
Calories	—	80	849	9.0
Protein	gram	0.3	26.4	0.28
Fat	gram	0.8	77.0	0.82
Carbohydrate	gram	20.0	27.7	0.29
Calcium	mg.	10	332	3.5
Phosphorus	mg.	14	716	7.61
Iron	mg.	0.4	6.7	0.07
Sodium	mg.	1.0	6.0	0.064
Potassium	mg.	152	1,098	14.9
Vitamin A	I.U.	120	0	0
Thiamin	mg.	0.04	0.34	0.0036
Riboflavin	mg.	0.03	1.31	0.014
Niacin	mg.	0.1	5.0	0.053
Ascorbic Acid	mg.	6.0	(Trace)	(Trace)

(Plus the following minerals, omitted from USDA handbook cited above):

Magnesium	mg.	10.4	378	4.0
Copper	mg.	0.02	1.7	0.018
Zinc	mg.	?	0.35	0.0037

Note: Also omitted from Agriculture Handbook No. 456 are a number of important vitamins that are known to be present in almonds in varying amounts. These include: biotin, vitamin B-6, folic acid, inositol, pantothenic acid, and vitamin E, as well as carotene, which the human body uses in manufacturing its own vitamin A. (For further details on the vitamin content of almonds, see "Almonds: Symbol of Life," by W.H. Church, *The A.R.E. Journal,* Vol. VI, No. 4, July, 1971.)

*Based on statistical information contained in Agriculture Handbook No. 4, *Nutritive Value of American Foods,* by Catherine F. Adams, USDA, Washington, D.C., 1975.

**This column represents supplemental data added by author, based on tested count of 94 almonds per 140 grams, measuring exactly 1 cupful. Statistical information on magnesium and copper obtained from *Nutrition Almanac,* Nutrition Search, Inc., John D. Kirschmann, Director; McGraw-Hill Book Co., NY, 1975 (paperback ed.). Information on zinc content in almonds from letter, California Almond Growers Exchange, 2/11/74.)

Table 2—A Comparison of Mineral Values, 2 or 3 Raw Almonds (Unblanched) versus 1 Medium Apple (Raw, Unpeeled)

Constituent	Unit of Meas.	ALMONDS 2 Raw Unblanched	ALMONDS 3 Raw Unblanched	APPLE (RAW) 1 Medium-size Unpeeled
Calcium	mg.	7.0	10.5	10.0
Phosphorus	mg.	15.22	22.83	14.0
Iron	mg.	0.14	0.21	0.4
Sodium	mg.	0.128	0.192	1.0
Potassium	mg.	29.8	44.7	152.0
Magnesium	mg.	8.0	12.0	10.4
Copper..........	mg.	0.036	0.054	0.02
Zinc	mg.	0.0074	0.0111	?

Another important aspect of the almond is its rich protein content, containing all eight of the essential amino acids (those that the body cannot manufacture for itself), plus several others. These are of vital importance to all cellular functions. And what of the relatively high fat content in almonds? It is 95 percent unsaturated. Twenty percent is linoleic acid, one of the essential fats the body cannot produce. Its role in maintaining healthy skin tissue suggests a probable link-up of some kind with whatever it is in the almond (probably a *combination* of factors!) that makes the almond a natural hedge against skin blemishes and tumors, according to the readings.

Then there are the vitamins. And here we must digress for a moment. Vitamins, it should be pointed out, never work singlehandedly. Rather, they are chemicals that function in partnership with hormones, enzymes, and many other substances—including the various mineral ions, of course. That is why the "vitamin" view of cancer therapy or prevention is an incomplete one and can be very misleading. Yet we would not deny that vitamins are an essential component. They are interlaced everywhere in the endless chain of fleeting chemical reactions taking place within us, converting food to energy and energy to cellular reproduction. The vitamins in the almond include, in addition to a fair level of riboflavin, an impressive amount of niacin. Niacin is one of the B-complex factors often mentioned in connection with cancer therapy, along with vitamin E. (Although present in the almond, vitamin E was omitted from the chart of nutritive values used by the compiler of the official USDA nutritional statistics, from which we drew our data for Table 1. Choline, another vitamin factor in the almond, falls in this same category.)

Finally, one more vitamin in the almond must be mentioned.

This is amygdalin. It has never been officially recognized, and so it is always ignored in any officially compiled nutritional handbooks. Amygdalin is also identified as Laetrile, or vitamin B-17, when extracted from apricot kernels or from bitter as opposed to sweet almonds. We had once supported the supposition that amygdalin might be synonymous with an unidentified "form of vitamin" mysteriously referred to in one of the readings that spoke about almonds. (659-1) However, there are some scientific arguments to unseat that supposition. Laetrile, as most readers know, is a widely disputed anti-carcinogen that has been associated with claims of cyanide poisoning in some isolated cases; it is normally used in combination with a total dietary approach to cancer—and not alone, which must raise some inevitable questions as to its real efficacy. In any case, it is believed that the cyanide molecule that makes Laetrile effective against cancer is *inactivated* in the amygdalin present in sweet almonds, apparently due to the absence of the fermenting agent, emulsin. If this medical assumption is correct, the amygdalin in our daily ration of sweet almonds is not only harmless but, it would seem, presumably useless, as well! However, another view of amygdalin has surfaced recently in the news.[3] It credits the benzaldehyde in this vitamin substance, rather than the cyanide factor, as the effective cancer-fighting agent. Yet it claims, paradoxically, that the benzaldehyde must be mechanically extracted and administered *directly* to the patient because the human body is incapable of extracting it by natural assimilative processes. It is a claim that is obviously open to dispute in some quarters, and will perhaps never be resolved to everyone's satisfaction! No matter. After all, it is the mineral constituents in the almond with which we intend chiefly to concern ourselves here. Some of these micro-nutrients appear to hold promising clues in our search for the almond's secret potency.

III

First, phosphorus. And there is more to say on this subject, perhaps, than on any other aspect of the almond. All of it is fascinating.

"Recent research," according to one source,[4] "has shown that phosphorus may be important in cancer prevention." This is not surprising. Why? Investigators have discovered a telltale symptom in cancerous cells: *low phosphorus counts.* We know that a proper balance of phosphorus, calcium and iron in the body is very important. Calcium aids in phosphorus absorption. Yet excess phosphorus hinders iron absorption. However, if calcium is present in sufficient amounts, it will combine with the phosphates and release the iron for use. It is interesting, in this respect, to note that the almond combines *all three* of these important minerals, and presumably in a ratio suitable for their ready absorption, if we may judge by this next excerpt from the readings:

The almond carries more phosphorus *and* iron, *in a combination easily assimilated* than any other nut. [author's italics] **1131-2**

Quite plainly, if the iron and phosphorus are in a combination that is easily assimilated, it can be safely assumed that they are in a compatible ratio with each other; and this must also be true of the calcium content of the almond. Yet we can see, in Table 2, that the ratio of phosphorus to calcium is approximately 2.2 parts phosphorus to 1 part calcium, whereas a healthy body should maintain a calcium-phosphorus balance in its bone structure of 2.5 parts calcium to only 1 part phosphorus—just the reverse of the almond's ratio. On the other hand, the phosphorus content in the soft tissues of the body, including the brain, is significantly higher than in the bones. More specifically, phosphorus metabolism in two of the seven endocrine glands—the pineal and the pituitary, in that order—is found to be *extremely high*.[5] This is an exciting discovery. Aside from their spiritual significance, as described in the Edgar Cayce readings and other sources of an esoteric nature, these two closely associated glands in the brain cavity play a vital role in hormone production. Research on the hormone melatonin, produced by the pineal gland, is still at an unsophisticated stage; but it would appear to cause "vivid visual imagery and hallucinations."[6] And although imbedded deep in the brain, the mammalian pineal is found to be "responsive to outside light," which may be attributed to the melatonin factor, perhaps, or to the nature of the gland itself. The precise biological function of melatonin is not yet fully understood by medical science, although students of the Cayce readings may be able to recognize a relationship with the activity of the so-called third eye or "single eye of service," which can be aroused in periods of deep meditation. There are numerous references in mystical literature to a deep blue, and sometimes a clear white, luminosity encountered in association with this center, which is located at a deep central point behind the brow.

Getting back to the almond, then, it is interesting to speculate on a possible connection of some kind between the high phosphate requirements of the pineal and pituitary centers and the high-level phosphorus found in the almond. *(Phos,* incidentally, is a Greek word meaning "light"![7]) It must be admitted that the human body's total needs for phosphorus far outstrip whatever can be supplied by ingesting only two or three almonds daily; and the same is also true of its calcium and iron requirements. But we intend to show that this is not too relevant. The phosphorus in a limited supply of almonds might be of a sufficient quantity and of just the right sort qualitatively to supply the *specialized* phosphate needs of the pineal and pituitary glands in their hormone-producing functions. Those functions, moreover, appear to affect the whole reproductive system. This indicates how proper nourishment to these glands, administered by way of the nutritious almond on a daily basis and in judiciously restricted amounts, might indeed be able to protect the body against the development of cancer or tumorous growths of any kind, as claimed in a number of the readings.

The question that currently arises out of all this theorizing is whether or not the physical body may possess some sort of collective intelligence, operating within its individual cells, that would enable it to assimilate and distribute phosphorus on a *selective* basis from the foods ingested, so that phosphates extracted from the almond could be directed to the pineal and pituitary centers, and not elsewhere. We answer, Yes. According to the readings, every cell is a universe within itself and knows its purpose. The individual and collective cells, therefore, exhibit intelligence, responding either to the Divine within or to its opposite. Diseased or disordered cells simply reflect the response of the body to contradictory and destructive patterns of human thought and behavior exhibited at the conscious or subconscious level.

It is of interest, at this point, to note that the German mystic, Jacob Boehme, who experienced illumination on a number of occasions while in the meditative state, employed an arcane term of his own invention, "the restoration of phosphorus," in connection with his unique description of the inward transformation process of spiritual alchemy. We know, moreover, that the raising of the kundalini force in deep meditation only reaches its fullest expression when it ascends to the pineal and pituitary centers. In the Cayce readings and commentary on the Book of the Revelation,[8] we find the pineal gland equated with the "Name," or the Christed Consciousness, and the pituitary center equated with the "Kingdom of Heaven." (Those who have opened this last center, in meditation, are the comparatively rare few who have experienced what Hindu saints refer to as *Samadhi* or what is sometimes referred to in the West as Cosmic Consciousness. It is a state of bliss.)

In a related vein, we discover that one of the early Gnostic sects—the Naasenes—borrowed from the Phrygians "the comparison of the Father of the Universe to an almond kernel, existing before all things and containing within itself the perfect fruit from which was to come forth an invisible child, nameless and ineffable."[9] This Naasene reference to a child, it seems clear, was to the coming appearance of the Christ. But in the original Phrygian version, according to C.G. Jung, "the Father of all things" was *Amygdalos,* or almond tree;[10] and the almond kernel, therefore, would appear to be a more proper representation of the invisible Son. All of this has an even deeper symbolic significance when we recall that enigmatic statement in reading 3180-3, which was probably alluding to the days of Noah and the Great Flood: "The almond blossomed when everything else died. Remember, this is life!" Is it any wonder, then, that the Old Testament writers ascribed sacred powers to the almond, from Aaron's magical rod to Jeremiah's compelling vision of the rod of an almond tree?[11] Finally, among the tomb decorations in a Gnostic sepulchre unearthed at Rome, circa 1930, was what appeared to be an illustration of the Christ as the "Good Shepherd," in a frame decorated with almonds.

So we can say, quite conclusively, that there exist some striking historical and legendary references to support our view of a very real relationship between the almond and the "Father/Son" synonymity of the pituitary and pineal centers. Such a relationship appears to have existed from the beginning.

On a final esoteric note, the fact that phosphorus functions as the body's major anion, or *negatively* charged ion, may be of significance in relation to the role of phosphate in the pineal and pituitary glands. (By contrast, calcium, magnesium, potassium and sodium all function as major cations, or *positively* charged ions.) During meditation, when the spiritual centers are attuned and are in a "negatively polarized" or receptive state, the negatively charged phosphate ions in the pineal and pituitary areas may facilitate the raising of the Christ Presence within us as a *positively* charged force, attracted to its polar "opposite." (One is reminded of that mystical term, "the marriage of the opposites," which was used so frequently by the ancient alchemists, who disguised the spiritual nature of their "work" under elaborate symbols!)

But all of this is purely speculative, of course.

Further on the subject of phosphorus and cancer research, there is an unconfirmed report out of Japan on the experimental use of the chemical element *luciferin* in the treatment of certain types of cancer.[12] Luciferin is derived from such bioluminescent organisms as the common lightning-bug, whose luminosity, in turn, comes from luminous bacteria in its abdomen. These bacteria are known to use riboflavin phosphate in light production. Interesting, isn't it? Whether or not there is a riboflavin-phosphorus bond in the almond remains an interesting question for the chemical researcher to resolve. If so, it is possible that this is the almond's mysterious "form of vitamin" referred to in reading 659-1. But because of the unconfirmed nature of the Japanese report, we can only mention it casually, in passing.

IV

Next we come to potassium.

A potassium deficiency is thought by some nutritional experts to be a contributing cause of cancer.[13] In fact, going a step further, Dr. Passwater cites "a very much deteriorated mineral picture" as a typical pattern in virtually all patients who have malignancies, even in the incipient stages.[14] But probably deficiencies in phosphorus and potassium are the most notorious. (Selenium, a trace mineral, may be a third in this category).

Potassium functions with sodium to equalize the acid-alkali factor in the blood. And this leads us to another interesting observation about almonds, which, unlike other nuts, have an *alkaline* effect. Perhaps the high potassium content of the almond is responsible. At any rate, potassium-rich foods are commonly included in nutritional therapy for cancer. And since cancer cells will take up potassium readily (provided that it is introduced in a manner that will facilitate retention), there is even a theory in some circles that by increasing the alkalinity of these malignant cells, potassium may aid in their destruction.[15]

To retain the storage of potassium in the cells, however, an adequate supply of magnesium is necessary. Magnesium not only promotes the absorption and metabolism of potassium and other minerals, but—like potassium—it also helps regulate the acid-alkaline balance in the body. Here, again, we find the almond containing this essential mineral.

The role of copper, one of the trace minerals in the almond, is somewhat controversial. It is toxic at high levels, but very useful in lower amounts.

This mineral is found in the almond at a ratio of about 5 to 1 over zinc, which would be dangerously high, and even fatal, if that same ratio prevailed in all of the other foods ingested. Fortunately, very few foods have a preponderance of copper to zinc. But the role of copper in connection with the other nutrients in the almond may require this higher level, since copper functions as a *brain stimulant*. And it may have a synergistic effect in combination with phosphorus, fueling and stimulating the pineal and pituitary glands. We know, at any rate, that copper is required for the synthesis of phospholipids. One of the places in the body where copper concentrations are found, not surprisingly, is in the brain. The recommended daily allowance of copper is established at 2 milligrams for adults; and since only 1.7 milligrams are provided by an entire cupful of almonds, there is obviously no risk of copper toxicity in a daily intake of just two or three almonds or less.

And, finally, what of zinc?

Probably more has been written about this trace mineral than any other, and it has been the subject of much intensive research. This is because it appears to offer a great deal of promise in many areas of nutritional therapy, and it is relatively non-toxic. But because of its rather restricted presence in the almond, we will not explore its uses or its literature in detail.

Zinc aids in the healing process. It also plays a key part in phosphorus metabolism, and its limited presence in the almond may serve to fulfill that specific function. At the same time, high intakes of zinc interfere with copper utilization, which will cause incomplete iron metabolism. The major function of iron is to combine with protein and copper in making hemoglobin.

In short, iron builds up the blood and increases resistance to stress and disease. We have already read that the iron content in the almond is in a combination with phosphorus that is "easily assimilated," so all is well.

V

In summary, we can only marvel at the intricacy and wisdom with which a Higher Intelligence appears to have designed the almond. It is indeed that "perfect fruit" of the early Gnostics. And more than that. The almond is a living symbol of life itself! In truth, it is an unborn almond tree—an "Amygdalos" sleeping. We can try to dissect it, to analyze and define its separate parts. We may learn a little, but we miss a lot. For a seed is a living, pulsating organism. It emits an energy field peculiar to its nature, and it has a vibratory rate to which it resonates continuously. Only the psychic self can discern these things. Yet they are there. And they are very real indeed. Then how can we hope to unlock the almond's secrets by a process of fragmentation any more than the essence of a man is to be found in an examination of his chemical components? Goethe was right: the whole *is* greater than the sum of its parts. It is as true of an almond seed as it is of Man himself. And it is true of God, whose divine seed we are.

FOOTNOTES

[1]An examination of the vitamin content in almonds was included in our previous article on the subject. See "Almonds—Symbol of Life," *The A.R.E. Journal,* Vol. VI, No. 4, July 1971.
[2]See readings 820-2, A-8; 5091-1.
[3]Report by Walter Cronkite, on cancer research in Japan; *CBS Evening News,* Jan. 29, 1979.
[4]*Nutrition Almanac,* p. 77.
[5]Research notes by Stephen Goranson, supplement to reading 1602-3.
[6]"Do Saints Really Glow?" *San Francisco Chronicle,* May 11, 1977.
[7]Goranson. See footnote #5 above.
[8]Extracted from the 281 series and published separately. *A Commentary on the Book of the Revelation,* A.R.E. Press, Virginia Beach, Va., 1973.
[9]*The A.R.E. Journal,* Vol. VI, No. 4, July 1971, p. 133.
[10]*Alchemical Studies,* p. 87.
[11]Numbers 17:1-8; Jeremiah 1:11-12.
[12]Paul Harvey news broadcast, KGO, San Francisco, Aug. 1977.
[13]*Nutrition Almanac,* p. 119, citing Rodale.
[14]Passwater, p. 183.
[15]*Ibid.,* p. 184.

BIBLIOGRAPHY

Adams, Catherine F. *Nutritive Value of American Foods.* Agriculture Handbook No. 456, USDA, Agricultural Research Service, Washington, D.C., 1975.

Ariola, Paavo. *How to Get Well.* Health Plus Publishers, Phoenix, Ariz., 1974.

California Almond Growers Exchange, Sacramento, Calif. Letter of 2/11/74 re: zinc content in almonds; also, "Chemical Composition of Natural Nonpareil Almonds" and other technical data, 1979.

Church, W.H. "Almonds—Symbol of Life," *The A.R.E. Journal,* Vol. VI, No. 4, July 1971, pp. 133-141.

Donsbach, Kurt W. *Minerals,* International Institute of Natural Health Sciences, Huntington Beach, Calif., 1977.

Doresse, Jean. *The Secret Books of the Egyptian Gnostics,* The Viking Press, N.Y., 1960.

Holy Bible, King James Version.

Jung, C.G. *The Collected Works of,* Vol. 13, "Alchemical Studies," Bollingen Series XX, Princeton University Press, 1970.

Kirschmann, John D. *Nutrition Almanac,* Nutrition Search, Inc., McGraw-Hill Book Co., N.Y., 1975.

Passwater, Richard D. *Cancer and Its Nutritional Therapies,* A Pivot Original Health Book, Keats Publishing, Inc., New Canaan, Conn., 1978.

Pfeiffer, Carl C. *Zinc and Other Micro-Nutrients,* A Pivot Original Health Book, Keats Publishing, Inc., New Canaan, Conn., 1978.

The Psychiatrist and Castor Oil Packs

Ernie Pecci, whose special concern is mental retardation, was one of the outstanding lecturers at the A.R.E. Medical Symposium. At his two Multipurpose Centers near Oakland, California, he has been working with castor oil packs applied to the abdomen. A recent letter from him states, in part: "In what I would call a major breakthrough, a University of California medical researcher wants to conduct some research studies on the use of the castor oil packs based upon our previous success. They are especially interested in investigating my hypothesis that 'minimal brain damage' is really an endocrine dysfunction which might be helped with the use of the castor oil packs. They have set up an elaborate EEG monitoring system which can be linked to computers which would indicate whether learning is really enhanced after treatment."

EDGAR CAYCE AND THE PALMA CHRISTI

by William A. McGarey, M.D.

The following article is composed of excerpts from a research paper (now an A.R.E. Press book entitled *Edgar Cayce and the Palma Christi)* which presents a study of the use of castor oil packs as suggested in the Edgar Cayce readings, and as observed in the practice of general medicine. Dr. McGarey found the readings to represent the largest body of information having to do with the use of castor oil packs as therapy.

His title comes from an exhaustive search into medical literature which produced a book published in 1918 by Douglas W. Montgomery, M.D. Dr. Montgomery wrote that castor oil was extracted from the seed of the *Ricinus communis,* sometimes known as the Palma Christi (the palm of Christ) because of its palmate leaf structure.

The first portion of the report includes a survey of the use of castor oil and some of its history—in industry, folk medicine, and as therapy. In this section also Dr. McGarey deals with physiology, emotions, functions and eliminations. A careful accounting is given of various kinds of incoordination—in the etiology of body sickness, and as pertaining to attitudes and emotions.

The second portion of the report shows the use of castor oil packs today, case histories, failures and successes, and physiological conclusions. The Editor

The Purpose of Castor Oil Research

Castor oil packs and their use on the human body occupy the central position of our study. Research has indicated that their use extends back in time to ancient Egypt, where castor oil was used therapeutically. We can see how these packs are related to parapsychology by studying their use in the readings of Edgar

Cayce—a man who could lie down and voluntarily enter a state of mind and body wherein his conscious mind was apparently not involved with what he was saying.

Cayce indicated that his entire autonomic nervous system was vitally active during this state, and that the unconscious mind was that portion which was seeking out and reporting the information found. Often this information came from the unconscious mind of the other person involved—and this would seem to direct us to the haunting thought that we know already what is wrong with our bodies. We just can't reach down into that unconscious mind (or is it the autonomic nervous system?) and obtain the knowledge that we would like to have.

Thus the seeking into the nervous system of man became proper here, since, in bringing together all portions of this study, the inferences in the Cayce readings cannot be ignored. And these state that castor oil packs seemingly have a relationship with the nervous system and most of the other systems of the body in aiding the body back to health.

This brings us, then, to the study of their use in the general practice of medicine, and the analysis, for whatever value may proceed from it, of 81 cases in my practice where individuals who had varying conditions of illness were treated through the use of these packs.

These 81 cases (of which only 8 are noted here) are a random selection and represent only a small fraction of the instances where we have used castor oil packs as the only, or as a coordinate, therapy for one condition or another of illness. Some of the cases in which I have been most impressed by the therapeutic efficiency of this tool are not included. A continuing effort is being made, however, to collect more data which—it is hoped—will provide statistically significant information that is not to be found in this preliminary report.

My object in presenting these cases in conjunction with the other information that has been presented is fivefold in its scope: (1) to stimulate interest in this therapeutic regime; (2) to show the exceptionally wide latitude of use that is possible with the castor oil packs; (3) to present and coordinate evidence that there is actual beneficial response in the human body to the application of these packs; (4) to discuss theoretical considerations relative to the action of the packs on the body; and (5) to begin to explore the validity of a unique understanding of physiological functioning of the human body, which is found in the Edgar Cayce readings.

Castor Oil Packs

Instructions for use:

Prepare first a soft flannel cloth which is two or three thicknesses when folded and which measures about eight inches in width and ten to twelve inches in length after it is folded. This is the size needed for abdominal application—other areas would need a different size pack, as applicable. Pour some castor oil into a pan and soak the cloth in the oil. Then wring it out so that the cloth is wet but not drippy with the castor oil. Then apply the cloth to the area which needs treatment.

Protection should be made against soiling the bed clothing by putting a plastic sheet underneath the body. Then a plastic covering should be applied over the soaked flannel cloth. On top of that, place a heating pad and turn it up to "medium" to begin with—then to "high" if the body tolerates it. Then perhaps it will help if you wrap a towel around the entire area. The pack should remain in place between one and one-and-a-half hours.

The skin can be cleansed afterwards, if desired, by using water which is prepared as follows: to a quart of water, add two teaspoons baking soda. Use this to cleanse the abdomen. Keep the flannel pack in a pan for future use. It need not be discarded after one application.

Examples of Case Histories

Case No. 8. A 33-year-old male accountant presented himself with the chief complaint of severe constipation for one month, associated with generalized abdominal distention. He gave a history of having had some degree of chronic constipation since childhood, with distention. During the month just past, he noted that laxatives only caused cramping, but gave him no real relief. Examination showed all findings to be within normal limits except for abdominal tenderness, most marked over both lower quadrants. There was no tenderness noted over the gall bladder area or over the pancreas. He had been treated in the past with contact evacuants, peristaltic stimulants, and cholagogue-pancreatic enzyme mixture. The diagnosis used here is constipation. The history is suspicious of pancreatic or liver-gall bladder malfunction. Full workup with x-ray and laboratory tests were not performed.

Treatment consisted only of castor oil packs in association with a low-fat diet. The patient cooperated well in applying the packs three days in a row each week, for one hour each time, for a total of seven weeks. Results were very satisfactory. The bowel movements became regular, once daily. The cramps disappeared, and the abdominal pain ceased. Examinations showed a normal abdomen with no tenderness elicited.

Response rated as excellent to single therapy.

Case No. 13. 75 years. This elderly widow was a resident of a rest home, and was seen because of a furuncle which had developed in the left axilla. She complained of much pain associated with the furuncle, which was not draining. She had been hospitalized many times, once earlier that year for surgical drainage of a furuncle in the right axilla. General health was poor and she had been an arthritic for many years. Examination of the local area showed much rubor and swelling in the tissues of the furuncle and surrounding it. Patient complained bitterly of the pain and was unable to move arm without much difficulty. No fluctuation could be found at that point. Diagnosis was, of course, furuncle of the left axilla.

No treatment was used with the exception of the castor oil packs which were used twice daily for 1½ hours for a period of 17 days. The tenderness and pain subsided within 2-3 days, and then the furuncle gradually cleared until it disappeared completely. There was no evidence of fluctuation having occurred at any time although the degree of tissue inflammation may have masked some of the signs which might otherwise have been observed. Thus there was no external drainage of material from this lesion at any time.

Response was rated as excellent to single therapy.

Case No. 14. This was an 11-year-old boy who liked to play baseball. He was struck by a batted ball over the right maxilla two weeks before being seen first in my office. The lump which developed in that area persisted and was growing gradually larger. Examination revealed an 8 mm. fibrous tumor of the subcutaneous tissue overlying the right maxillary prominence, which was tender to palpation. X-rays were negative for fracture. Diagnosis was fibrohematoma of the subcutaneous tissues.

Treatment suggested was use of a castor oil pack to that area for 45 minutes daily, to be used for a period of two weeks. The family cooperated very well, and reported that the tenderness subsided in the first few days, and the size of the nodule gradually became less. When he was examined in two weeks, the tumor was difficult to find because of its size, which was then perhaps 2 mm. in diameter, and the consistency was softer. Treatment was stopped, and the nodule then disappeared over a period of time.

Response was rated as excellent to single therapy.

Case No. 15. A 37-year-old male, married grocer, developed a urinary infection three days before being seen in our office on 7/1/65. Symptoms were low back pain and dysuria. His past history revealed two episodes of renal calculus, in 1959 and again in 1963, and occasional upper respiratory infections. Examination showed tenderness over both costovertebral angles, and urinalysis performed on that date showed albumen and the centrifuged specimen to be loaded with white blood cells. The patient was given a sulfa-azo dye medication and the infection cleared within a week, when the medication was stopped. Infection recurred two days later, but ten days of treatment did not do the job, and the patient was seen on 7/19/65 with original presenting symptoms. Diagnosis was cystitis and pyelo-nephritis.

Treatment with castor oil packs was begun on 7/19/65 while continuing the other therapy. They were used over the renal areas of the lower back all night long for five days. The aching subsided after the first night, recurred briefly on the third day and then disappeared again. Examination on the fifth day showed absence of tenderness over the left C.V.A., and only minimal tenderness over the right. The medication was cut to half dosage, the packs were continued for another 10 days after that and the patient continued to complete clearing signs, symptoms and laboratory evidence of infection.

Response was rated as excellent to combined therapy.

Case No. 16. A 51-year-old housewife was in the midst of marital difficulties which had progressed to divorce proceedings when she was seen in our office with specific complaints of depression, nervousness, episodes of numbness, anorexia, nausea, abdominal cramps and distention, associated with much mucus in her stools which were loose in character. These had all existed over a period of about two months, although she gave the history of having had symptoms of colitis over the past five-year period. Her physical examination showed a normal blood pressure of 100/70, and local findings of generalized abdominal tenderness, most marked in the epigastrium. There was hyperperistalsis present. Diagnosis for this survey purpose was mucous colitis. (It is evident that there was a great deal of stress present here and tension, depression, etc., but this was not evaluated as was the colitis, so was not used as a diagnosis.)

Treatment was already being used: a colitis diet and two types of ataraxics plus an anti-spasmodic for smooth muscles. These were continued, and castor oil packs were added to the regimen, being used three times a week for 1½ hours daily over a period of four weeks. During this period of time, the cramps subsided, mucus no longer appeared in her stools and the bowel movements became more normal. Peristalsis decreased. The packs were discontinued, and sometime later most of the symptoms recurred.

Response was rated as good to combined therapy.

Case No. 18. 11-year-old schoolboy. The boy experienced onset of abdominal pain with low-grade fever and vomiting while visiting relatives in California. The physician consulted stated that he had symptoms of appendicitis, gave him an injection of penicillin and advised the parents to go home immediately to seek further care. He was brought to my office the next day with the history that he had continued to have nausea, anorexia and abdominal pain. His temperature at that point was 98.6 degrees, and examination revealed tenderness in the right lower quadrant with positive rebound tenderness. There was no rigidity, no masses palpable and peristalsis was present. Diagnosis was acute appendicitis.

The mother did not want surgery unless necessary. Since a critical point requiring surgical intervention had not arrived, I elected to watch and wait, instituting the use of castor oil packs again without the use of the heating pad. The patient was put at bedrest, given only ice chips by mouth, and, with the pack on continuously, he remained comfortable the remainder of that day. He spent a good night, feeling much better in the morning. At that point, his nausea disappeared. On examination, his tenderness was only minimal, and the rebound phenomenon was gone. He was given a full liquid diet, bedrest was continued, and the packs were kept on continuously. On the second morning of this therapy, patient was completely asymptomatic. The packs were used two to four hours that day and a light diet was prescribed. Although there were no symptoms and the boy was impatient to be completely active, he was given the packs twice on the third day for one hour each. At that point, his diet was normal and he resumed full activity with no further therapy.

Response was rated as excellent to single therapy.

Case No. 30. This was a 40-year-old married secretary, who was seen with common warts on her right index finger, a condition which had been present for several months. The largest was 8 mm. in diameter. Diagnosis was verruca vulgaris, right index finger.

These were treated by applying a band-aid to the warts on the finger, the bandage portion being first soaked in castor oil. This was worn continuously, being changed once or twice a day for a period of two months. At the end of that period of time, the warts had completely disappeared.

Response was rated as excellent to single therapy.

Case No. 36. 42-year-old housewife, registered nurse. This is perhaps the most unusual case in the series, and I refer to it fondly as "the case of the curly hair." This woman presented herself with the request that I check her blood pressure. She stated she had hypertension and she believed it was due to taking a contraceptive medication for a period of time and to much tension to which she had been subjected. Blood pressure was first discovered to be elevated less than six months before her first visit to our office. Her chronological story began, however, some 16 months before this first visit. She started taking, at that point, contraceptive pills, which she continued for a total of 13 months. After being on the medication for two months, a series of very traumatic events occurred in her family. After four months on the medication she developed noticeably increased nervousness. At five months she experienced a 21-hour uterine hemorrhage that was difficult to stop. At the six-month period, she noted cramps in both legs. At the nine-month mark, when her personal tension was also at its height, she developed swelling of the left calf, and the cramps in her legs became at times excruciating.

Also, when she washed her hair, she noted that for the first time in her life she could not make the hair develop a suds. She changed shampoos three times to no effect, and the beauty parlor met with the same results—no sudsing. At this point it was noted that her blood pressure was elevated. Her legs continued to bother her severely, and the veins in her legs were distended until, after 13 months on the medication, she stopped it of her own accord. Her gynecologist did not believe that the medication was causing her trouble, according to her account. When she stopped the medication, her veins became normal and the cramps in her legs stopped bothering her. Her blood pressure remained elevated, however; she remained tense, and her hair retained the remarkable non-sudsing quality. The texture of her hair was poorer and it would not curl as well as it did before all this started. She then saw an internist who examined her thoroughly and could find nothing wrong with her except the elevated blood pressure, which he did not think was caused by tension or by the medication. Within a few weeks after this, she came to our office. Examination revealed a blood pressure of 180/110 to 160/98, with no other abnormal findings.

She was treated for three months with conventional medication for hypertension, and the blood pressure remained constant, not responding. Then, about six months after she had stopped her medication, she complained of palpitation and tenseness again, and I was ready to begin use of the packs. Her diagnosis recorded for purposes of this study were hypertension and oral contraceptive reaction.

Therapy was continued with the hypertensive medication. The only other therapy advised was abdominal castor oil packs, applied three consecutive nights of each week for three weeks in a row, duration 1½ hours each treatment. The third pack each week was to be followed by oral ingestion of one ounce of olive oil. The patient followed the instructions, and reported when she returned in three weeks that after one week's treatment with the packs her hair sudsed like it hadn't in nearly ten months, and there was a marked improvement in the texture of the hair and in its curling qualities. She noted no other change in symptoms.

Response was rated as excellent to single therapy for the oral contraceptive reaction; poor to combined therapy for the hypertension.

Physiological Conclusions

In this summary statement, I shall attempt to accomplish several ends, while effecting a comprehensible relationship between a number of physiological concepts which have been dealt with in this study. We should deal more concretely with the theory of the manner in which castor oil packs work. We should try to bring a relationship between the use of this mode of therapy as advised by Edgar Cayce, and the manner in which it became effective as a tool in the practice of medicine.

Cayce seemingly approached the human body from within, looking at it intimately, seeing it function, even to the manner in which one nerve cell bridges the gap to its synaptic partner, and seeing the substance which allows this to happen. He was able to see the symptoms in a body, and what we might call a disease process coming into being from a single source—which may be very distant and difficult to pin down as a cause, as far as we are concerned.

In the 81 cases in which the castor oil packs were used as a principal method of treatment, we have approached an understanding of the body more from the outside, so to speak. This outside approach is what derives from an acquired understanding using the findings of this physical world as guideposts. It might be termed a conventional approach—at least *more* conventional than found in the readings.

If we can perhaps correlate these two groups of data, these two sources of information which have been presented here, it may well lead us into a better understanding of the human body as a whole, a goal truly worth striving for.

This study is being concluded with the hope that it will invite more research of a nature which will produce more acceptable evidence, answer more of those as-yet-unanswered questions, and do it in a manner that will bring closer together the understanding of the various natures of man, whose makeup at this point seems to be body, mind and spirit—three elements whose manifestation is as a unit and whose three parts are equally valid, important and whole.

How does castor oil as a pack act in the human body? How does it bring into being a beneficial effect in body tissues? Among other things, we observed that the packs, when used in the 81 cases, produced the following results: brought a peaceful sensation to the abdomen, affected beneficially the autonomic nervous system; induced changes in the lymphatics, relieved bodily stress, restored curly hair (!), apparently affected ganglia and plexuses, cleared up infections, aided pregnancy, benefitted systems (e.g., genito-urinary), and affected beneficially areas of the body such as the pelvic organs in toto.

Cayce, in his readings, gives us ideas relative to the effects that castor oil has in the body when applied in such a manner, but the understanding is not easy to come by. I would like to use two references first, then comment on them. The first was an answer to a question about a psychic experience a 33-year-old woman had; and Cayce brings the castor oil into this discussion, relating it significantly, I think. The second extract is from a reading four years earlier given the same woman who had been applying psychic information from Cayce and was highly desirous of becoming pregnant.

This was an interbetween emotion, or—as indicated—a partial psychic experience.

Consider that which takes place from the use of the oil pack and its influence upon the body, and something of the emotion experienced may be partially understood.

Oil is that which constitutes, in a form, the nature of activity between the functionings of the organs of the system; as related to activity. Much in the same manner as upon an inanimate object it acts as a limbering agent, or allowing movement, motion, as may be had by the attempt to move a hinge, a wrench, a center, or that movement of an inanimate machinery motion. This is the same effect had upon that which is now animated by spirit. This movement, then, was the reflection of the abilities of the spirit of *animate* activity as controlled through the emotions of mind, or the activity of mind between spirit *and* matter.

This was a vision, see?   1523-14

Then, for the betterment of the general conditions as a whole, it would be well that much of an analysis be given; that the conditions which are existent be thoroughly understood from a psychological, pathological and physiological standpoint.

These are not meant to be mere terms, but indicate rather the boundaries of the various changes which have taken place, and are taking place, in this body.

In other words, then:

The body, as an entity, is experiencing the result of the mental attitudes of the body through a given period. Thus, psychological conditions have brought, do bring, their effect upon the general systems of the body.

Hence, these are—as the name indicates—a creative, an activative force through the mental and the physical conditions of the body.

Thus there should be, then, the realization that organs and their functionings have become aware, or conscious, of their activity, their function within the system.

While as yet this is not a true or full conception, there is the awareness and the awakening of those influences within the system . . . 1523-8

In the first selection, Cayce is saying that the castor oil, when applied, is active as that which allows the acting together or coordination between the *functioning* of organs in the system. He indicates elsewhere that in his terminology any acting part of the body is an organ, so the nervous system, muscles, etc., would all qualify as organs. The oil assumes this relationship of being the *means,* perhaps, by which the organs function together only when the activity of the body as a whole is considered, it being directed by higher intelligence. Thus, when one performs an action, oil allows the body to coordinate and act. (Oil, of course, is found within the body, and in a condition of health, the packs would not be needed anyway.)

The above extract seems to be saying that the oil acts upon the mind forces, or acts to allow the mind forces in the body to become active in producing better coordination between parts of the body *and* in bringing the spirit into closer communication with the body through these mind forces. Somewhat like putting oil on a wheelbarrow's rusty axle. The wheel will then work in better coordination with the barrow, but it takes the one directing to move it and let the two parts of the wheelbarrow perform better than before their individual functions. The spirit, then, is enhanced in its motivation of the body, through the improved coordination brought about within the parts of that body by the castor oil in its application and action.

The second extract, of course, shows that Cayce believes that consciousness, mind quality, awareness of a particular sort, exists within the very tissues, cells and organs of the body. Thus he sees the castor oil as bringing to the body a closer working together and cooperation between the minds of these tissues or organs, as the body relates to the spirit which motivates it and gives it life.

He does not say in what physical way the oil brings this about, but we can see how such a concept would explain the results which have been attained in practice. Perhaps the autonomic nervous system provides the physical counterpart of the "activity" that Cayce mentions as occurring between the functionings of the organs; and oil, in its vibratory essence, becomes the "nature" of that activity, bringing about a better coordination and a resultant bodily function that spells healing to the individual. How can such a concept be simply explained? Cayce involves us with the spirit of life, so we become even more than just body and mind, if he is correct. In any event, this is a credible idea which does give understanding to results obtained, and perhaps gives us a better idea of what sort of conditions might be benefited by such therapy.

What part is played here, then, by the lymph, which has occasioned so much comment thus far? This must be discussed in a summary form, as it relates particularly to the function of the autonomic nervous system, for these are closely related and important one to the other.

Cayce sees the lacteals as that anatomical portion of the body which makes it possible for the body to take values from the food and to prepare these values in such a manner that they can be used to revitalize and bring back to life, so to speak, all the tissues—the entire system—of this same body. Moreover, he sees the Peyer's patches as creating a "globular" substance which is carried by the lymphocytes to the contact points between the "sympathetic" and the cerebrospinal nervous systems, which occur in the spinal cord, or the sympathetic ganglia, which lie anterior to the spinal column. This substance is necessary to form a contact between these two systems, and lack of proper contact brings sometimes physical disorders, sometimes mental derangement that varies from very mild to critically serious in its degree. He infers that this lack of contact is a true lack of relationship (in one cell or millions of them) between the physical consciousness and the "soul and spirit forces"—what we may perhaps call the unconscious mind. The implications of this, of course, are rather widespread and drastic, and leave much suggested which cannot be elaborated upon here.

This same area just mentioned—the spinal cord relationship or connection to the sympathetic ganglia—is often the site of difficulty, which Cayce explains as a "lesion" which forms, due to injury or depletion of the system in certain foodstuffs or nutritional needs, or perhaps through stress situations in life. The following selection demonstrates one manner in which the readings see this lesion coming into being, and indicates that it in turn causes trouble to the system.

In the beginning, then, or cause, or seat of the trouble, we find that there was that in the system that produced a depletion to the physical resistance. During this period there

was an injury, or a subluxation, to the 9th and 10th dorsal vertebrae. In the recuperation, in ease, the body formed a lesion to meet the needs of the condition.   943-1

This philosophy of function in the human body, as becomes gradually apparent in study, would have us understand that these lesions which are formed, then, become the etiology of other troubles throughout the body—through imperfect transmission of impulses from the higher brain centers to the general areas of the internal workings of the body, which are controlled autonomically by the ganglia thus affected. We have seen this in the selections already quoted. Then a function such as the liver performs is affected, and coordination between the liver and perhaps the kidney as a portion of the elimination of the body becomes a problem. The patient may then develop a frequency or irritation without evidence of infection. Through the disturbance to the liver, the digestion may be affected, and then, in quick order, the assimilation of needed food qualities is limited, the energies of the body suffer, and the nervous system is affected through the lack of substances given to the lymphatic system and subsequent inadequate lymphocytes and again the "globular" substance. So one can see that, in the same manner that "man is not an island," the organs of the body do not stand alone. They are units only in being parts of a larger unit.

Even those many qualities of the world outside of oneself are sensed in such a manner that it becomes effective as an influence on the functioning of the body as a whole. Sounds, colors, tastes, odors, the "feel" of something—all these are shunted through the autonomic nervous system, in which manner they become as influences to the organs and tissues of the body as part of their individual consciousness, as these same sensations make their way to consciousness of the whole individual. Even the lesions which occur in the body, as Cayce describes them, become associated with the energies of perception and sensing. In the instance that follows, the lesion is not apparently associated with the spinal cord-ganglion relationship, but rather is one of those created in the abdominal cavity, which may be the type conceivably created by lymphatic disturbance and inadequate lymphatic drainage from a given site. (This does not seem to be quite clear, yet—at least in my studies of the readings.)

Q-4. What happened, a few months ago during the headache,

when something seemed to pop in my head—since which time the attacks haven't seemed to be as severe?

A-4. There is the coordination between the nerve systems, as we have indicated, at the area where the medulla oblongata enters the lower portion of the brain, see? At that period when there was such a severe attack, there was the breaking of a lesion in the *abdominal* area. This *sounded* through the sympathetic nerve system, *producing* the condition in the head itself. For, as was indicated, it appeared to go *through and out* the head.

1857-1

The emotions, response within the individual to conditions outside the body in relationship to other people, self's evaluation of self, all bring about within the body a disturbance that often sees certain areas affected according to the emotions experienced. But the balance within the body organs and body systems becomes disturbed, elimination is hindered, intake of food is associated with turmoil, and the beginnings are seen of body sickness through just the mechanisms which have been here only lightly touched upon.

The readings frequently mention that the circulatory system (as related to the autonomic) is a site of disturbance in various parts of the body. These relationships were not made clear in the study just completed, nor were those which bring together the efficacy of the castor oil packs in pelvic diseases and the sacral parasympathetic supply to these organs.

Much in the way of physiologic function, as seen by these readings which Cayce gave for over forty years, becomes shifted into the first levels of understandability, as serious study is given to portions of the readings. The rationale of castor oil pack therapy begins to become apparent. And few, if any, contradictions show up in the rather startling number of words which flowed in such a strange manner from the lips of a dedicated man and the reaches of an unconscious mind.

We begin to see that it is not so strange that a castor oil pack can be applied to the abdomen, and in one person a vaginitis is cleared up; in a second case a fecal impaction causing intestinal obstruction is relieved; in a third a threatened abortion is rendered into a normal pregnancy; in a fourth a cholecystitis is cured; and in a fifth, after ten long months, the hair is made to curl and shampoo to suds once more. Unless physiologic factors were at work that we do not wholly understand, these things could not be.

Cayce, whose work on these readings ceased over twenty

years ago with his death, would undoubtedly agree that this last extract would speak to these strange results from a strange therapy.

For, what is the source of all healing for human ills? From whence doth the body receive life, light, or immortality? That the body as an active force is the result of spirit and mind, these coordinating and cooperating, enables the entity to bring forth in the experience that which may be used—or the using of the abilities of whatever nature. Each soul has within its power that to use which may make it at one with Creative Forces or God. These are the sources from which life, light, and the activity of body, mind and soul may manifest in whatever may be the active source or principle in the mind of the individual entity . . .

There are, then, as given, those influences in the nature of man that may supply that needed. For, man in his nature—physical, mental and spiritual—is a replica, is a part of whole universal reaction in materiality.

Hence there are those elements which if applied in a material way, if there is the activity with same of the spirit and mind, may bring into the experience of each atom of the body force or cell itself the awareness of the Creative Force or God. It may only rise as high as the ideal held by the body-mind.

Hence there is the one way, the source. For in Him is all life, all health, all mind, all knowledge and immortality to the soul-mind itself.   3492-1

Those who are receptive in their nature will benefit most from the packs. Why is this? Because being receptive is being as the little child. He has faith without even knowing why, and so accepts all things as being the will and the graciousness of God acting in his life. And the peace comes to him, throughout the whole of the earth—His earth.

Healing may really be peace—a peace that comes to rest in the body, that is a reflection of the "peace that passeth understanding." We see it come to the body much as peace is allowed to come to the earth: a nation here and a nation there. When we find real peace in the earth, we may see a state of health having come to all bodies.

IPSAB—An Herbal Remedy for Gum Problems

by Tom Johnson and Carol A. Baraff

Numerous readings recommend a solution called Ipsab as a treatment for the gums and teeth. It is not known where the name originated—possibly it was coined by Edgar Cayce's source of information. In Cayce's day at least, Ipsab was not a commercial product.

Many readings prescribing it also gave directions for making it, but these formulas varied somewhat. In a few instances it is stated that the finished product should be a paste, but the majority of cases suggest a liquid. If desired, a paste may be easily made by adding salt in sufficient amounts to the liquid.

The Ipsab formula requires prickly ash bark, salt, calcium chloride, peppermint and iodine. Salt acts as an astringent, shrinking the gum membranes between the teeth so that the other ingredients can reach these areas. The primary active ingredient is prickly ash bark. This was known to the American Indians as "toothache bark," and Cayce referred to it by the same terms.

In many cases Ipsab was suggested simply for general upkeep of teeth and gums:

Using, then, for the teeth and gums, to strengthen same, those properties as found in that combination [Ipsab] as has been given for such conditions through these forces. 257-11

Some local attention [to the teeth] is needed. The natural tendency of a disturbance in the circulatory forces to the sensory organs, as indicated, is to make for a lack of the proper circulation through the gums and to the portions of the teeth themselves.

If the solution known as Ipsab is used to massage the gums occasionally, it will make for a *strengthening* of the areas and a preserving of their usefulness. Once or twice a week this would be thoroughly massaged into the gums, and will make a great deal of change in the gums and the teeth.

Do that.   987-1

Do use Ipsab as a massage for the gums and it will make a great deal of difference with the teeth, the breath and the general activity.   3598-1

We would use same [Ipsab] not upon cotton, for this body, but upon the finger use it and massage; not only the gums where the teeth are but where they are not! And we will find that the stimulation to the activities of the throat itself, to the salivary glands, to even the tonsil area, will be materially aided by the activity of the combination of the calcium with the iodine in same, as well as the antiseptics that arise from the vegetable forces in same as combined with sodium chloride.   569-23

Ipsab, in diluted form, was recommended for the developing teeth of babies. The following readings were given for a one-year-old and a nine-month-old child, respectively:

Also, during this period of the formation of the teeth, keep sufficient quantities of iodine in the food values for the body, as well as calcium, and so forth. It will be found that a massage of the gums occasionally with those properties known as Ipsab will be helpful ... as these processes are carried on through the activity of the thyroid operations in the body.   314-2

Q-2. Are teeth forming normally?
A-2. These are very good. We would find that a weakened solution of Ipsab for the gums would tend to relieve the pressure and make for normalcy in the salivary glands, as well as strengthening the tissue in mouth. This should be reduced at least half, and the gums massaged with a tuft of cotton with same. This also adds to the amount of saline, calcium and iodine, for the activity of the glands in mouth and throat.
                                                                     299-2

Ipsab seems to be especially effective in treatment of bleeding or receding gums and for treatment and prevention of pyorrhea. In one reading Cayce stated that some element in the prickly ash bark destroyed the germs that cause pyorrhea. Ipsab was also prescribed for trench mouth and other types of gum problems:

Q-1. What can I do about pyorrhea condition in my teeth?
A-1. Use Ipsab regularly each day and rinse mouth out when
it is finished with Glyco-Thymoline.   5121-1

The receding gums and those tendencies towards pyorrhea
would be allayed by the consistent use of Ipsab as a massage
for the teeth and gums. Also these should be treated, some
locally, with the dentist's paraphernalia [and also]—the small
wads of cotton saturated with the Ipsab and applied in the
areas where the conditions are indicated at the base or edge of
the gums.   3696-1

This will *purify* and make for such a condition as to assist in
correcting the trouble where there has been the softening of
the teeth themselves—or the enamel on same.   1026-1

On the Matter of Warts

Bob Brewer says: "I always use castor oil as an aid to the
elimination of warts. I use the electric needle on the wart itself,
and then during the entire healing period, a castor oil soaked
bandaid is used." He has had no recurrences. Bob Forbis, on the
other hand, had a different story. He speaks from his
experiences as a dermatologist in San Diego. He tells me that:
"Warts are driving me right up the wall! I have been handing
out the castor oil and the castor oil-beeswax (90%-100%)
ointment to a large number of patients with a variety of
different results. The thing that keeps you going is the once-in-
a-while good result of any kind of a wart—flat, plantar,
condyloma, accuminata, or ordinary vulgar warts. The
problem is that I just don't consider the percentage of good
results above the placebo level of success." This reminds me of
the report in the *British Medical Journal* about the physician
who "bought" warts from little people. The kids loved it—the
doctor paid them sixpence for a wart and told them that it
would be gone in three days. And it was. His suggestion was
strong medicine. I have tried this, using dimes, but have had no
success. On the other hand, my own percentage of wart
treatment with castor oil is about fifty percent. Perhaps my
patients have a stronger castor oil consciousness.

GLYCO-THYMOLINE

by Cecil Nichols

This paper was prepared for the Medical Research Division of the Edgar Cayce Foundation, Inc., Virginia Beach, Virginia, in January, 1966, with conclusions and recommendations.

Purpose and Data

This paper is based upon the study of 193 Edgar Cayce readings wherein Glyco-Thymoline was prescribed in one or more ways.

Glyco-Thymoline is manufactured by Kress and Owen Company and, according to the manufacturer's literature, is to be used as a "treatment for mucosity (abnormal excessive mucous secretion)" and for several other types of external application.

The Edgar Cayce readings recommended Glyco-Thymoline for use in the following additional areas: as an internal antiseptic with water; as a pack; and as an eye-wash.

Analysis of these 193 readings shows no pattern of treatment given for specific ailments concurrent with the administration of Glyco-Thymoline, although in a broad sense many other types of therapy were prescribed.

It must be borne in mind that these physical readings were given for specific people having specific ailments. These ailments were not always clearly defined either in the readings or in the background material. For this reason no attempt has been made to analyze statistically the data collected from the readings.

Glyco-Thymoline as an Internal Antiseptic

The readings leave little doubt as to why Glyco-Thymoline is recommended to be taken internally. Consider the following extracts:

. . . **[take] three drops of Glyco-Thymoline in water before** retiring at night . . . The Glyco-Thymoline acts as an intestinal antiseptic of an alkaline nature . . .   3104-1

. . . take occasionally small quantities—eight to ten drops—of an *intestinal* antiseptic, such as is seen in that of Glyco, or that as is found in any of those that are of the *alkaline* reaction. Such as may be seen in forms of those of the pepsins, that keep the system the more alkaline in the stomach's reaction proper.
                                                                              99-5

The key words here seem to be "acts as an intestinal antiseptic of an alkaline nature." In fact, the foregoing statement, either direct or paraphrased, appears in 76 of the readings studied which prescribed internally administered Glyco-Thymoline.

. . . use an alkalizer for the alimentary canal . . . each day take three or four drops of Glyco-Thymoline internally, in a little water. Take this for sufficient period until the *odor* of same may be detected from the stool. This will purify the whole of the alimentary canal and create an alkaline reaction *through* the lower portion of the alimentary canal.   1807-3

The readings emphasize the necessity of an acid-alkaline balance within the human body.

The diet should be more body-building; that is, less acid foods and more of the alkaline-reacting . . .
Keep closer to the alkaline diets; using fruits, berries, vegetables, particularly that carry iron, silicon, phosphorus and the like . . .   480-19

Apparently the Glyco-Thymoline was administered internally to help bring the over-acidified body back into balance. There seems to have been nothing magical about the action of Glyco-Thymoline itself, as other commercial formulations completely different in chemical composition were sometimes offered as substitutes.

Q-2. What intestinal antiseptic should be used . . . ?
A-2. That that is alkaline in its reaction, Lavoris or Glyco-Thymoline.   653-1

In some cases studied, the dosage of internally administered Glyco varied from as low as 2 to as high as 15 drops of Glyco-

Thymoline in water. The dosage was apparently in accord with the degree of over-acidity to be corrected. The body was apparently judged to have had enough Glyco-Thymoline when the odor of same was detected in the stool.

Experimentation with internally administered Glyco-Thymoline is not recommended except under the supervision of a qualified medical doctor, because one may become over-alkalized.

As indicated, keep a tendency for alkalinity in the diet. This does not necessitate that there should *never* by any of the acid-forming foods included in the diet, for an overalkalinity is much more harmful than a little tendency occasionally for acidity. But remember there are those tendencies in the system for cold and congestion . . . and cold *cannot—does not—*exist in alkalines.   808-3

Glyco-Thymoline as a Pack

It is abundantly apparent throughout that the readings recommended Glyco-Thymoline packs for a great variety of cases. There was, however, some variation in the way the pack should be applied. In some cases an unheated pack was recommended. In other cases heat was applied over the pack, and in some cases a specific type of heat was used.

The following are extracts from the readings which illustrate the construction of the Glyco-Thymoline pack as well as the modes of applying heat.

On the throat apply three to four thicknesses of cotton cloth saturated with Glyco-Thymoline, full strength, normal temperature—not heat applied.   1112-9

. . . place over the area on the spinal column two thicknesses of heavy cotton cloth saturated with Glyco-Thymoline. Place over this for five to ten minutes a hot water bottle . . . and let it be pretty warm.   4045-1

Each day for one hour we would apply Glyco-Thymoline packs over the areas across the hips, throughout the ileac plexus. Use three to four thicknesses of cotton cloth saturated in Glyco-Thymoline. Apply heat. Also use the Glyco-Thymoline packs around the knee, but *do not* apply heat here. But *do* apply heat over the sacral area. These are to aid in eliminating the accumulations there, through assisting the system to absorb poisons.   3281-1

At times a salt pack was recommended as a means of heating the Glyco-Thymoline pack as the following reading shows:

Over this [the Glyco-Thymoline] pack use salt heat—not just a bag of heated salt, but sew the salt into a container—quilted, as it were. Heat this in the oven and apply over the Glyco-Thymoline pack, instead of using an electric pad. Preferably use iodized salt; not so hot as to burn, but let the body lie upon or over the pack.   987-5

Packs in general seem to be in keeping with standard medical practice as evidenced by the following quote from *The Merck Manual*, 8th edition, p. 1488: "The object of applying moist heat to the body is to ease pain, supply moisture, and promote circulation, muscle relaxation, or wound-drainage.

"It may be given in the form of soaks or compresses, which also serve to wash away any discharge that may be present. The principal solutions employed are water, isotonic salt solution (0.9%), magnesium sulfate (3-6%), and boric acid (3%), but many other medicinal substances are also recommended as dressings . . . Moist compresses, using cotton gauze, flannel or towels, may be kept at the desired temperature by overlaying with one or more hot water bottles and enclosing the whole area in oilskin or cellophane; this also will prevent rapid drying out of the compress. Electric pads must not be used in this manner because of the danger of electric shock in the presence of moisture."

The following reading seems to speak the same language as the above quote from *The Merck Manual* as to the usefulness of a pack:

. . . there should be a systematic series of osteopathic adjustments. However, each time before these adjustments are made—which should be twice each week—we would relax the area to be adjusted by applying heavy packs of Glyco-Thymoline. Use three or four thicknesses of cotton cloth saturated with warm Glyco-Thymoline and apply for at least an hour to an hour and a half, the day before the adjustments are to be made. Let these packs extend over the lumbar area and all of the sacral area, even to the end of the spine. Apply heat over this, not too much but sufficient to cause these properties not only to relax the body but to be absorbed into those areas. Thus the osteopathic corrections, when administered the next day, will relieve these tensions and make for those tendencies towards a better coordination and a better alkalinity in the eliminations. Thus the activity to the kidneys will be aided, also of the bladder and organs of pelvis, as well as the activity for the whole body.   3157-1

Various External Uses for Glyco-Thymoline
In addition to the categories covered above, the Edgar Cayce readings recommended Glyco-Thymoline for various other external uses. These external applications appear clear-cut and are presented as reading extracts.

Q-1. What should be done to relieve my eyes?
A-1. Bathe these with a weak Glyco-Thymoline solution. Use an eye cup, and two parts of distilled water (preferably) to one part of the Glyco-Thymoline. This irritation is a part of the kidney disturbance that has come from the upsetting in the digestive forces.   3050-2

Q-6. What is the cause of my throat filling with a black mucus?
A-6. The inhalation of those properties about where the body works. But with the gargling each evening and morning with Glyco-Thymoline, this will aid, and if a little of it is swallowed it will not hurt.   1688-9

. . . at least twice each week—especially following the periods, but twice each week at other times—we would use a vaginal douche with Glyco-Thymoline as the antiseptic. Use only the fountain syringe in taking these douches. Use at least a quart or two quarts of the water, body-temperature, and put two tablespoonsful of Glyco-Thymoline to each quart of water used.
. . . with the douches as a purifier for the organs, we should bring about normal conditions.   2175-4

. . . have a good hydrotherapist give a thorough, but gentle, colon cleansing; this possibly a week or two weeks apart. In the first waters, use salt and soda, in the proportions of a heaping teaspoonful of table salt and a level teaspoonful of baking soda dissolved thoroughly to each half gallon of water. In the last water use Glyco-Thymoline as an intestinal antiseptic to purify the system, in the proportions of a tablespoonful to the quart of water.   1745-4

Conclusion and Recommendations
It has been the author's attempt throughout the course of this

paper to quote extracts from the quantity of readings studied which are representative of the complete body of information contained therein relating to Glyco-Thymoline.

Where exceptions to the rule were encountered they were so noted.

The most important point gained from the many readings studied is the prime importance which is attached to the acid-alkaline balance within the human body, a point which medical science seems to consider of little consequence.

Administered internally, Glyco-Thymoline was apparently for the purpose of regaining balance in the overacidified body. A slower (but probably surer) way of doing the same thing is to correct the diet.

It is recommended that a qualified medical doctor be engaged to study the effect that the acid-alkaline balance (pH) in the stomach has on the assimilation and elimination of foods and on the presence (if any) of disease in a body. Obviously, the M.D. is the final authority.

These extracts are not presented as prescription for treatment of diseases but rather are selected to indicate the point of view taken on the particular problem of the individual who sought psychic information at that time.

Hearing Problems

When we look at deafness from a broader view, we see physical disturbances as immediate apparent causes, but psychological and perhaps spiritual influences involved as basic background factors. Modern psychiatry recognizes that hearing problems in the older person are often caused by that person becoming "tired" of listening to others, and an actual physical condition develops because of emotional reactions. Deafness has often been described in the Cayce life readings as having been karmic—a result of one turning a "deaf ear" to someone's needs at a critical time in a past life.

OUR EXPERIENCES WITH THE RADIO-ACTIVE APPLIANCE

by Barbara and Brent Parisen

Since our introduction to the Cayce material six years ago, we have been striving toward our ideal—to "live the Life" and to attain that perfect balance of body, mind and spirit so necessary for becoming more perfect channels of blessings to others. Consequently, in keeping with this ideal of attunement and service, we have had to make significant changes in our diet, exercise habits, attitudes, relationships, and life style in general. After prayerful consideration, we employed various attunement aids, such as wearing the lapis lazuli stone, studying music, taking Atomidine, and using the radio-active appliance—all of which are recommended in the Cayce readings. We have found all of them helpful; however, the radio-active appliance, when used in conjunction with prayer and meditation, has proved to be of enormous assistance. Application of this device has brought a multitude of benefits which we would like to share with you. It is our hope that after reading about our experiences, you will feel moved to investigate it as another aid to your own attunement.

The radio-active appliance is mentioned in the readings some 450 times and was recommended for problems ranging from adhesions to epilepsy to paralysis to vertigo.[1] In fact, Cayce stated that the "radio-active [appliance] plain [without the use of solutions] is very good; good for everybody!" (631-2), "especially to *rest* tired businessmen, overtaxed ladies . . ." (1800-16)

According to Cayce, the appliance is unlimited in its use and its range of benefits, for not only does it make the body physically more fit by bringing about better circulation, assimilation, relaxation and elimination,[2] but it actually aligns and rejuvenates the body's mental and spiritual forces along with the physical by bringing about "a better coordination in the cerebrospinal and sympathetic systems." (593-1) No other medical device has this unique capacity to restore that complete physical-mental-spiritual balance!

In addition to an improved physical condition, use of the appliance, the readings promise, will bring new self-awareness and greater understanding. To one inquiring individual Cayce said: ". . . there will be periods of exciting experience in the spiritual and mental self." (5199-1) He advised another to pay attention to the unfoldment of "the real subconscious self" in dreams which occur during the period of the appliance applications. (911-2)

In light of the physical benefits and these spiritual promises (which in our experience we have found to be real), the radio-active appliance is truly priceless!

"Those vibrations from the appliance given are not just as talismanic conditions," says reading 957-3, "nor are they that which operates through the imaginations of a body, but when properly compounded or constructed these correspond with the laws of physics . . ." The radio-active appliance is a simple battery formed of carbon steel.[3] The battery becomes "electronized" (activated) by the ice water into which it is placed; then, when attached to the body by the copper and nickel plates, it partakes of the body's vibrations.

Every cell in the body has an electrical vibration, *is* vibration. However, through injury, reaction to internal or external forces, or lack of proper elimination or equilibrium, some cells become deficient in the vital energy they need for reproducing themselves and maintaining the necessary balance in the system. Other cells contain an abundance of vibratory energy. The appliance receives the vibrations of the body's excess electrical energy through the positive (copper) lead and, via the negative (nickel) lead, returns that life-giving, equalizing energy to those parts of the body deficient in this energy. See the illustration below:

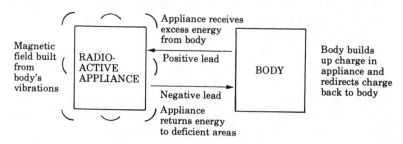

Magnetic field built from body's vibrations

RADIO-ACTIVE APPLIANCE

Appliance receives excess energy from body

Positive lead

Negative lead

Appliance returns energy to deficient areas

BODY

Body builds up charge in appliance and redirects charge back to body

The result is an "equilibrium in the human body [which enables the body] to relieve any tension . . . caused in the deficiency or over proficiency of any electronic agent as is set forth by any of the organisms as are found in the human body." (1800-4) This equilibrium "enables the quieting, then, from within, and allows the forces to become predominant that are constructive to *vitality* in system." (957-3)

No other vibrations are involved except those produced by the body. The appliance acts only as a generative magnet, building up a magnetic energy field from the body's electrical vibrations, which are then discharged back to the body, "[revivifying] portions of the body where there is a lack of energies stored." (3105-1) "There is nothing in the appliance of itself," said Cayce. "For, know, as you are told in the Book, in the law—all that is within heaven and earth, as well as hell, is within the body of the living individual." (3119-1) The appliance acts "as an equalizer and would only act in that same force wherein *normal rest* to the body becomes recuperative powers for same." [italics ours] (1800-4)

"Normal rest," it must be noted, may be compared to the trance state from which Cayce gave this information, for occasionally when he reached this state he would say that his body had assumed its "normal forces." If this is the case, very few of us have ever rested normally!

One does not need a doctor's prescription in order to use the machine; also, a doctor is not needed to apply it to the body, since it is easy to attach.[4] Handicapped persons, however, may need some help. For specific ailments, use of the appliance was often recommended in combination with other treatments, such as osteopathic or chiropractic manipulations, massages, oil rubs, herbal remedies, colonics, packs, hydrotherapy, and exercises. But these treatments should not be administered to the body while the appliance is attached. And if other Cayce-recommended appliances are being used, such as the wet-cell or violet ray, they should be used "out of phase" with each other, as reading 1268-2 states: ". . . we would not use the appliance during the strong use of the other influences..."

Nor should there be a great deal of mental activity, such as conversation or the study of problems, during the time of application. Rather, we are instructed to use this time to analyze ourselves and our relationship to God, to examine purposes and ideals, study Scripture, and read the Bible—not as a history or a book of axioms to be followed, but as a personal message—especially Genesis 1:1-6, Exodus 19:5, Deuteronomy 30, John 14-17, and Psalms 1, 23, 24 and 91.

This time should also be a period for prayer and meditation, "not only for the removal of the disorders but that the purposes of the body and mind may be used for creative, constructive purposes . . ." (3632-1) We should pray "for the body to be used in the service for others, and not others in a service for the body." (4069-1) In other words, it is not enough that we merely contemplate these things while the radio-active appliance is attached. We must make a personal, practical application of these truths throughout our daily lives.

Know . . . that with the changes wrought [by the appliance], these are not to be made for self-aggrandizement, self-indulgences, but that the spirit of truth, of good, of love, of patience, of reproduction, may be fully accomplished...
1389-1

We are even admonished to beware of selfish purposes. If we want help only for ourselves and are not willing to use our renewed health for aiding others, we should not even use the machine.

Each and every soul then that would touch these, in any form or manner, [must] dedicate their lives to a service for humanity! And *those not willing to do so, give it up!* [italics ours]
1800-28

Thus, it is primarily this attitude of selfless purpose that, along with the aid of the machine, brings the greater healing results. We must be patient and persistent, and not use the appliance haphazardly, for this "will do no good at all!" (569-23) We must be sincere, careful not to apply the machine as rote. We must be prayerful, asking that *"The Father of light and mercy and truth, create in this body that as will bring the perfect coordination of the members of the body itself, that the soul may manifest in a perfect body."* (1314-2) We must be grateful for the opportunity to re-establish balance in our system, which brings us a greater desire to know God's will and the strength to carry it out.

You can't use the radio-active appliance and be a good "cusser" or "swearer"—neither can you use it and be a good hater. For it will work as a boomerang to the whole of the

nervous system if used in conjunction with such an attitude.
1844-2

We must be "a man (or woman) after God's own heart," "humble even as He."

If we are willing to dedicate our lives to His service and persist with the discipline called for in using the machine, we will be beautifully rewarded. The following describes what we have experienced in our personal use of the (plain) radio-active appliance. Our findings verify many of the claims the clairvoyant Cayce made for the machine.

We discovered that with using the machine some benefits came about immediately, while others appeared only gradually. Some were obvious health changes—improvements definitely brought about by the use of the appliance; others, more subtle changes, could not be easily attributable to the machine alone, because we were also meditating regularly, following a natural, nutritious diet, and exercising daily.

With the very first application came immediate relaxation. We just wanted to curl up and go to sleep! Cayce did say that the appliance ". . . will put the body to sleep . . ." (1845-1) and that within a few minutes of using the machine drowsiness would occur. "There will possibly occur no feeling from the use of the appliance, except the feeling of being sleepy." (4023-1) In fact, when we do sleep with the appliance attached, we sleep deeper and wake up fully rested and raring to go! ". . . the body may rest much better when it sleeps." (434-1) With regular nighttime use, we have discovered that we now require from one to two hours less sleep. Sometimes Brent awakens at three in the morning ready to start the day. (So much for the appliance as an energizer!) And that sluggishness that sometimes hangs on even after a long night's rest is gone. "This, we find, will throw off that of the heaviness . . ." (327-1)

Since using the appliance, we feel more "put together" inside—more "in order." There is a wonderful sense of well-being, a deep, internal peace, especially during the day following a night's application. "These forces will . . . make for the abilities for the body to quiet self throughout." (1192-6)

The appliance has improved our circulation. I especially have been made aware of this, for there is more color in my face and I no longer suffer with cold hands and feet. "This will relieve that tendency of cold feet, that tendency of the poor circulation in the extremities . . ." (326-1)

Brent believes the machine has helped to correct his metabolism. It has made him more aware of the effect of certain food combinations (which Cayce talks about in his readings on diet). Working with that new insight while using the appliance, he has lost 17 pounds from his 5'11" frame without dieting and has remained at the reduced weight of 158 pounds for the past six months. Brent believes this is a case of the one helping the other—a mutual assistance—though Cayce did say the appliance would bring about improved metabolism and restore one to his proper weight. ". . . create a better metabolism and catabolism in the system . . ." (688-1) "The use of the radio-active appliance keeps nearer the normalcy as to weight..." (877-18)

Cayce also claimed that the radio-active appliance would sharpen one's memory, and we have found since using it that our memories have improved. We remember things at the most appropriate times; we don't have to hunt mentally for the right words with which to express ourselves during conversations; we retain more of what we read; and we remember our dreams more often and in greater detail.

Our dreams have become more lucid—often we know what the dream means while dreaming it or immediately upon awakening. Shortly after I began using the appliance, I had two consecutive ESP dreams, a type which previously I had dreamed only rarely. Our recent dreams show that we are taking charge of our lives: More and more often we find ourselves in the role of teacher, guide, helper, healer, even exorcist! It is our feeling that this leadership quality emerges as a natural consequence of being in balance; as we become more balanced, we are less preoccupied with self and more attentive to the needs of others.

And the more balanced we become physically, mentally and spiritually, the more closely attuned we become to the Universal Consciousness. As any meditator knows, this communion with the Divine Forces naturally brings an increase in guidance, enlightenment and inspiration. Among our recent blessings from using the appliance in conjunction with daily meditation have been the many revelations received concerning certain Biblical truths, especially those pertaining to the significance of the life, death and resurrection of Jesus the Christ. We have also received much insight into some personal karma, including an awareness of the lessons to be learned and how they are to be learned, plus a keener sense of the purpose of our present incarnation. In addition, we are shown how we can better help our loved ones, and are accordingly presented with more opportunities to be of service to them. Keys to diet-related discomforts, solutions to car problems, and ideas for stories and articles—along with the creative energy needed to bring these newly inspired projects to fruition—have been received.

But the most remarkable benefit derived from using the machine has been our change in attitude. The balance brought about by the radio-active appliance seems to have created a greater determination within us both to learn, to grow, to overcome. We are possessed with a tremendous drive to work, to do the things we must do, to do what He would have us do. Since we have used the machine, the outward circumstances of our lives have changed very little, but inwardly life has gotten easier because acceptance and patience come easier now. In fact, it is much easier to express all of the fruits of the spirit. There *is* effort, but the decision to choose right or good in favor of wrong or evil is easier because of the greater resolution to grow closer to our Father-God! This is without doubt the greatest blessing brought to us through the use of the radio-active appliance—this ambition to walk more closely with our Elder Brother, the Christ, along the path to our Father's house.

FOOTNOTES

[1] See the booklet *Two Electrical Appliances Described in the Edgar Cayce Readings* by Edgar Evans Cayce (A.R.E. Press, Virginia Beach, Va., rev., 1969, #63(P), $1.00) or the Circulating File—available to A.R.E. members only—*Appliance: Radio-active (Impedance Device)*, for the complete list of conditions and diseases mentioned in the readings in which the appliance was recommended for treatment.

[2] Reading 311-4 states: ". . . would the assimilations and the eliminations be kept nearer NORMAL in the human family, *the days might be extended to whatever period as was so desired . . .*" (italics ours)

[3] Instructions for manufacturing the appliance are given in the aforementioned booklet and Circulating File. See footnote #1.

[4] Instructions for general use and care of the appliance are given in the booklet and the Circulating File mentioned in footnote #1.

BALANCE—An End to the Common Cold

by Emory Michel

One of the most important requirements for complete participation in life is good health. Without it, a person can find himself unable to cope effectively with life's troublesome times or to derive full enjoyment from the smooth periods. Unfortunately, for precisely these reasons many of us seem to court disease. Illness can be used as an excuse to avoid facing our problems, or as a device for fulfilling a subconscious desire to cloud with suffering what would otherwise be the pleasant interludes; thus we often choose to ignore even the elementary measures that would keep the body in its best working order.

The common cold is one ailment that frequently proves convenient to contract. Medical science has provided very few clues as to the cause or cure of this condition; a host of remedies, from onion soup to Va-Tra-Nol to massive doses of vitamin C, have come into vogue from time to time, but none seems to have provided lasting effectiveness. Man is still in need of a widely available way of controlling this pesky disease, so that the vital energy currently being lost to it can be saved and constructively used.

One effective method of combating the cold seems to have been popularly overlooked. The psychic diagnostician, Edgar Cayce, who was often asked about a treatment for this disease, gave advice which never varied from the simple approach shown in this example:

Q-2. What can I do to build resistance against head colds?
A-2. Keep the normal acidity and alkalinity, by occasionally taking the test with litmus paper—both from the urine and from the spittle. Use the blue litmus, see?

When there is the inclination for acidity, use any of the sodas or their derivatives (citrocarbonates) as would make for producing a better balance. Thus we will find *the colds will be eliminated*. [author's italics] 1100-20

Can it really be so simple? Numerous individuals reported such advice was helpful when applied. Elaboration appeared in many other readings, such as the following:

Be mindful with the diet, that there are not acids; for colds and congestions arise from acid conditions in the system. Not so much starches. More of the fruit and vegetable juices, or fruit and vegetables in bulk.   307-7

In one reading, 480-19, the even broader suggestion was given that general immunization against contagious diseases was linked to the acid-alkaline balance of the body fluids.

A suggestion of the tremendous value of this simple technique for improving general health was given in a reading for a 35-year-old woman:

Q-6. Please give some general rules that will help this body to keep in a healthier condition.
A-6. . . . A general activity for a body in much of a normal condition is to keep the acidity and the alkalinity in a proper balance. The best manner to indicate this is to test the alkalinity or acidity of the body through the salivary glands or through the salivary gland membranes, or by taking the litmus paper in the mouth. This also may be indicated through the urine.

. . . if it is indicated in the salivary glands that there is an acidity, then take a small quantity of citrocarbonate. If the acidity is indicated through the kidneys, or from the urine itself, then drink a little of the carbonated waters . . . [bottled] Coca-Cola . . . *or* use a little of the watermelon seed tea. Either of these would tend to make for a balance.

Then if the proper balance is kept in the diet as indicated— twenty percent acid-producing to eighty percent alkaline- producing—as the conditions are for this body, its age, its temperament and the like—we should keep near normal.
                                                         540-11

The use of commercial antacid (alkalizer) compounds makes balance control quite simple when our system is temporarily off. For longer terms:

The foods, then, would be altered to meet that as would be found by *testing* the salivary reactions; litmus paper, yes—and we would find the body would, in three to five weeks, respond . . .   5456-1

Not awfully fast, but a simple way to know what change is needed!

In addition to our foods, the air around us also influences this acid-alkaline balance. Recently the acid condition of rain water has been reported to be on the increase. The Cayce information suggested testing for atmospheric (smog) effects on our body fluids:

> ... the climatic surroundings in the present especially, with such conditions as arise from the atmospheric pressures and the ladening of same with those influences that would tend to irritate especially the respiratory system—it would be well that the body check on itself occasionally as to the alkalinity, or acidity of the system. **1100-27**

The advantage of having a simple, direct system for measuring the effect of smog on our body system seems obvious. Instead of waiting to see if we are affected, we can measure our acidity with paper and use the appropriate treatment.

Before we go on to consider all the positive values the control of acid-alkaline balance can give, a warning about becoming over-alkaline is in order. This advice was given in a psychic reading about dietary practice:

> It is necessary, to be sure, that a certain amount of acid is kept in the system. An over-alkaline condition is much worse even than a mild acidity; for an alkaline reaction easily dissolves certain tissue, while an acid condition usually attempts to create the effluvia about the lymph circulation as to reduce acidity. **437-6**

Another example of this warning was found in reading 3390-1, given for a person whose body was weakened because the digestion and distribution conditions were severely unbalanced. The simple paper control test was again given as the best indication of the steps to be taken in regaining health.

In the following reading, a good general dietary formula was given for keeping the body fluids neutral:

> In the food values, then, keep a well-balanced diet that is nerve and blood building, and body building, but not those that would make for too great an excess of those forces that make for an excess of flesh. Leave off some of the starches. Keep the

proteins. Keep a well balance for all those foods that carry a well balancing of all food values, or those that make for the activities that produce the vitamins, or vitalities, or vitale, for the various functioning organs. Keep an even balance in the acidity and alkalinity of the body. It would be well were these tested occasionally, both from the spittle and from the urine, so that these show as to whether they are kept near to a normal neutrality in the system.   256-3

To a chemist, a neutral balance between acid and alkali is shown by a pH of near 7.0. Numbers above this value indicate an alkaline state; those below, acidity. For example, a pH of 6.0 would require the addition of alkali to become 7.0.

The readings contain many explanations of how various foods and combinations of foods affect acid-alkaline balance. While each body has its own unique dietary requirements for achieving balance, and many of the readings' recommendations were given to correct certain conditions in the systems of specific individuals, several guidelines that would prove valid for just about everyone can be formulated. Study of the Cayce material indicates the following general classification:

Acid Formers
1. Combinations of meats or fats with sugars or starches
2. Combinations of starches with sweets
3. Combinations of different starches, or too much starch
4. Combinations of acid fruits with starches
5. Cane sugar as compared to beet sugar, brown sugar, saccharin or honey
6. Candy before meals
7. Smoking before meals
8. Vinegar or acetic acid
9. Benzoate of soda (a food preservative)
10. Unbalance in elimination (constipation)

Acid Neutralizers (Alkali Formers)
1. Energetic activities
2. Orange juice plus lemon juice (mixed in a ratio of 4 to 1)
3. Grapefruit juice plus lime juice (mixed in a ratio of 4 to 1)
4. Grape juice
5. Pineapple juice
6. Cantaloupes grown in the neighborhood
7. Raw vegetables (in the ratio of 3 that grow above ground to 1 below ground or to 2 pod-type vegetables)

8. Combinations of stewed fruit with cereals (citrus juice should not be taken with cereal)
9. Lemon juice in tepid water about 30 minutes before breakfast
10. Citrocarbonate

This list is neither complete nor absolute for any one person. It is meant to demonstrate the combinations of foods that were given in the Cayce readings that might be helpful to someone attempting to control the acid-alkaline balance. The information must be verified by each individual. Much valid information is documented in various dietary systems, but it is important for each person to know what works for him. The ease of checking acid-alkaline balance by using a colored-paper test appears to provide a practical monitor system.

Laymen will find an excellent documentation of the individuality of each human digestive system in Dr. George Watson's "Nutrition and Your Mind." In a series of experiments by a research team, relationships between body fluid content, acid-alkaline balance, and the metabolic efficiency of interacting intermediate products were defined. In relating the individuality of dietary needs to each person, it was demonstrated that an excellent diet for one person was, in effect, a starvation diet to another, because of its action in the specific area of the physical mind. Subsequent controlled tests with a large group of mentally disturbed individuals were impressively successful in either improving or essentially curing severe mental cases. Balancing the metabolic efficiency for each, based on monitoring the blood pH (acid-alkaline balance), was a key factor in the treatment.

The individuality of the relationship of each human's physical condition and function with his mental and spiritual aspects receives prominent emphasis in the Cayce material:

... spirituality, mentality, and the physical being are all one; yet may indeed separate and function one without the other— and one at the expense of the other. Make them cooperative ...
307-10

When we fail to control this cooperative system, a physical reaction can be the warning signal of impending disturbance:

Few bodies there be that work themselves out. Not all rust

out, either. It is confusion that causes the greater disturbance in a physical body . . .   307-21

It is sincerely hoped that this information may serve as a guide in lessening confusion and achieving greater balance and harmony in the lives of those searching for a more abundant existence. It is in such a spirit that the Cayce information was provided:

. . . giving to the general public or to its peoples in many lands that which will show how that as there are added to the body-physical the elements of the soil in their proper ratio, these bring to the balanced mental and physical reactions the necessary forces for keeping the moral, the mental, the soul, the spiritual balance in the individual. And thus this is given out . . .   826-5

The following excerpt is even more explicit about the importance of achieving a broad dissemination of understanding:

Unless those activities among men are the aid for the greater number, rather than for the class or the few, they must eventually fail.   826-2

Finally, we hope that all may realize the purpose and importance of this effort to communicate a system which can help control the health of the physical body. In its relationship to our whole self, our physical being has a proper place, as given here:

As the body is the temple of the living God, preserve same in that way as of a sacred trust; that His spirit, His will may work through thee . . .   307-17

Author's Note

This writer's initial discovery of the desirability of the neutral acid-alkaline balance recommended in the Cayce readings came a few years ago; this was during or shortly after a period of suffering through a miserable head cold, followed by a chest cold. The disease had come in spite of years of good health while practicing Hatha Yoga techniques of body discipline. This apparent failure in my discipline had a very disturbing effect, inspiring a determined effort to find a system more adaptable to my active mode of living. The Cayce information showed me the way. Since I had been trained as a chemist and was professionally active in chemical process controls, the idea of controlling the pH, or acid-alkaline balance, of the body fluids was a premise immediately acceptable to me. Because of its inexactness, litmus paper was found unsatisfactory, however. The use of more recently developed and more readable acid-alkaline control papers was discovered in an extended personal test to be a more acceptable method of determining the body's pH.

Several ground rules were established for accurate control of measurements on saliva. Saliva placed on pH control paper in air gave erratic color changes. When pH was measured by placing the control paper under the tongue, the small flow of saliva produced by mild pressure of the tongue for just under 10 seconds gave reproducible readings of the acid-alkaline balance (pH). Assessment of the color of the pH control paper strip has to be made as soon as possible after the oral (under the tongue) test, so that the color change which occurs in air will not affect the reading.

This technique is easily mastered, but its success depends on using good judgment. Immediately after eating or using liquids, the accuracy of the saliva test is affected. Fair saliva test accuracy is obtained 15 minutes after rinsing food materials from the mouth with water. It appears to take three to four hours for the full effects of the assimilation of foods, medicines or the like to be reflected in the saliva test.

Changes in diet and physical activity levels may take several days or weeks to demonstrate their effect on saliva acid-alkaline balance. Only when such changes become regular and normal activities should their effect on body fluid pH be accepted as adequate for a well-balanced body. The acceptable pH range was found by my study to be 6.5-7.0.

Once a suitable balance for your system and life style has been found, it may occasionally be upset because of unanticipated changes. Such upsets can be diagnosed with the pH control test and balance can be quickly restored, before disease settles in to take its toll. The use of recommended amounts of widely marketed antacid compounds will often suffice for immediate treatment of over-acid test indications, until a normal pH pattern can reassert itself. A study of suggested foods given here, or of the more complete lists to be found in numerous diet and health books, should be considered by those who encounter difficulty in adjusting their acid-alkaline balance. Chronic problems should receive the attention of a cooperative physician. A tendency to overtreat with commercial antacids could affect the natural body forces which normally neutralize excess acid.

Rub Out Mosquitoes

Many massage oils were described in the Cayce readings; perhaps this is because massage was given as a therapeutic modality more often than any other type of therapy. From Quebec, Canada, comes an interesting story about one of these massage mixtures:

"I would like to tell you about a discovery I made, just by coincidence. Last summer . . . I used to prepare the solution prescribed by Edgar Cayce, a beauty aid for the skin (the peanut oil, olive oil, rosewater and lanolin mixture). Since I have a sensitive skin towards sunburns, I prepared it and used it as a suntan lotion all over my body . . .

"We used to spend the weekends in the Laurential hills, north of Montreal. The mountains are very beautiful, except for the unbelievable amount of black flies and mosquitoes. Needless to say, they manage to destroy any hopes of a trouble-free sunbath. Within minutes we were beleaguered by literally thousands of them. Everyone in our group was bitten awfully except a friend and myself . . . (we used the lotion) . . . Not *one* bite. This news might not be important to city dwellers, but . . ."

I would agree with my Canadian friend that those susceptible to insect bites might find this adaptation of the massage mixture beneficial. The exact formula, taken from reading 1968-7, is: peanut oil, 6 ounces; olive oil, 2 ounces; rosewater, 2 ounces; and lanolin (dissolved), 1 tablespoonful.

SKIN PROBLEMS:
Concepts from
the Readings
by Tom Johnson

The cosmetics industry as a whole has experienced an average growth rate of 10% per year during the past fifteen years. This extensive use of cosmetics shows that most of us are concerned with our physical appearance and the measures we can take to keep our skin in good condition.

A search through readings for people with skin disturbances reveals that Cayce placed great emphasis on the importance of internal conditions as a cause of complexion problems. The readings indicate that a large percentage of skin problems were a result of superficial or capillary circulatory disturbances often caused by poor assimilations, eliminations, glandular misfunctioning, and/or spinal misalignments and impingements.

Q-9. What is the cause of the skin eruptions that I have so frequently, and kindly give me a cure for same?
A-9. It has been given. These are a part of the circulatory disturbance, and as the eliminations are set up and as there are the coordinations between the forces in the body itself that make for a coordinant reaction in all portions of the eliminations, we will find these disturbances being eliminated. 603-3

Q-3. What causes the palms of my hands to be hard and dry, and at times to form little water blisters?
A-3. The poor circulation, and the lack of the activities or coordination between the glandular system and the eliminations. 1533-1

Q-2. What has caused recent increase of hair on lips, and what should be done to remedy it?

A-2. This, again, is from an inactivity and the allowing of overactivity in certain portions of the thyroid gland. For, this is the portion, in its balance, that keeps the body-forces in balance, adding to or taking from the system that to aid in the growth of hair, of nails, and in keeping an equilibrium. So, with the corrections of these conditions, and there being then better indications and the correct flow of this glandular secretion, these should gradually disappear. For these conditions use only such things as to correct the system, not any mechanical or chemical forces to remove these, see?

2582-1

Q-1. Is the condition [that I have] athlete's foot, as termed by the doctors?

A-1. Rather as indicated; and this is almost *always* the condition where there is what is termed as athlete's foot or where the locomotaries are disturbed. That is, an impingement. Here we find it below the locomotary centers proper, yet not sufficiently low to disturb the circulation in the upper portion of the body—but to make only external applications will not heal the conditions here. Then, it may be said to be the *symptoms* of athlete's foot—but reaches farther than this.

Q-2. What produced this condition?

A-2. First an accident or injury to that portion of the body, where the repressions in the circulation affected the lower extremities. Then the character of the shoe or, more specifically, the dye in the stockings worn. And then the addition to this of infection from external forces—fishy in its nature.

477-1

Exercise and adherence to the rules of diet were recommended as ways to improve the assimilations and eliminations as shown in these two extracts from readings for women suffering from skin disturbances. The first was for a 43-year-old woman; the second, for a 19-year-old girl.

Q-2. Can you suggest any treatment for dryness of hands and skin?

A-2. . . . The better change should come within from the better assimilation of that eaten, which will be found to be more improved by the exercises of stretching arms above the head, or swinging on a pole would be well. This doesn't mean to run out and jump up on a pole every time you eat, but have regular periods. When you have the activities, do have these exercises, for they will stimulate the gastric flow and let that eaten have something to float in . . .

2072-14

Q-4. Please outline a proper diet for me.

A-4. As indicated, do not use fats or highly seasoned foods, but those that tend to be more of an alkaline nature and the better for the system. No large quantities of sweets at any time, especially of cane sugar, but rather sufficient of that necessary to keep proper digestion ...   563-4

This would be well to be remembered by all:

Few germ formations, or none, that injure or cause distress in the form of neurotic, neuritis or arthritic conditions, or any form of skin eruption, may come when a system is tended toward alkalinity!   306-3

Cayce often advised people with skin problems not to depend on cosmetic preparations to solve their problems, since such preparations, while perhaps temporarily relieving the symptoms, cannot bring permanent cures.

Q-9. Is there not a treatment or method that might be used for the removal of blackheads from the face?

A-9. The general building up of the body forces and the establishing first of correct coordination or eliminations. These will gradually be removed.

There might be used bleaches, or cleansing creams, but these would eventually give more trouble than the blackheads are causing in the present. Get to the basic conditions of these, as being accomplished through the use of the fumes, the rubs and now the Violet Ray.   2072-9

Q-6. Can anything be done for pimples and breaking out of the skin?

A-6. The exercise and the diets are better than lotions or applications, see?   1771-3

Stimulation of the superficial circulation (the blood vessel network in the extremities and below the surface of the skin) seemed to be frequently recommended advice for keeping the skin in a healthy condition.

Q-3. What cosmetics would be best?

A-3. Don't depend upon cosmetics to clear or purify the skin. The cosmetics should be rather as an aid to keeping the superficial circulation in portions of the face and hands in bettered condition.   5271-1

This stimulation could be accomplished in several different

ways. Massage with oils was often recommended. The most usual combination was a mixture of peanut oil, olive oil, and lanolin. Many A.R.E. members are familiar with the following reading given in 1942:

> For making or keeping a good complexion—this for the skin, the hands, arms and body as well—we would prepare a compound to use as a massage (by self) at least once or twice each week.
> To 6 ounces of peanut oil, add:
>
> | | |
> |---|---|
> | Olive Oil | 2 ounces |
> | Rosewater | 2 ounces |
> | Lanolin dissolved | 1 tablespoonful |
>
> This would be used after a tepid bath, in which the body has remained for at least 15 to 20 minutes; giving the body then a thorough rub with any good soap—to stimulate the body-forces. As we find, Sweetheart or any good Castile soap, or Ivory, may be used for such.
> Afterwards, massage this solution, after shaking it well. Of course, this will be sufficient for many times. Shake well and pour in an open saucer or the like; dipping fingers in same. Begin with the face, neck, shoulders, arms; and then the whole body would be massaged thoroughly with the solution; especially in the limbs—in the areas that would come across the hips, across the body, across the diaphragm.
> This will not only keep a stimulating [effect], with the other treatments as indicated [hydrotherapy, massage and osteopathy] taken occasionally, and give the body a good base for the stimulating of the superficial circulation, but will aid in keeping the body beautiful; that is, as to any blemish of any nature. 1968-7

A mixture such as the preceding is known as an emollient. This is a cosmetic substance designed to lubricate, soften, and protect the skin against moisture loss. Cosmeticians often recommend emollients for people with dry skin problems.

The most unusual thing about this particular preparation is the peanut oil base. Almost all liquid emollients on the market today are based on mineral oil or castor oil. Olive oil, lanolin, and rosewater are all widely used in cosmetic formulas, although rosewater today is made synthetically.

The soap most frequently recommended in the readings seems to be Castile or Castile-based soap. At the time the readings were given the strict definition of this soap was one made from olive oil and caustic soda. The word "castile" comes from the Castile district in Spain, a large olive-producing section. Today, most Castile soaps include a varying amount of other fats, partly due to the high cost of olive oil.

Another item occasionally mentioned is the Boncilla mud-pack. It is apparently another way to stimulate the superficial circulation.

... about twice a month ... we would have the [Boncilla] mud packs; face and neck, and across the shoulders, and upper portion about the neck; especially extending over the area of the thyroids—as an astringent and as a stimulation for a better circulation throughout the system.   1968-3

In the cosmetic world, the Boncilla pack would be usually prescribed for oily skins. As an astringent it serves temporarily to firm and tighten the skin. In another reading Cayce suggested that the Boncilla mud had a type of chalk that was especially beneficial. Of course, cosmetic mud is not the same as ordinary mud.

Overall, the readings advise us that external applications will not cure the blemishes caused by internal problems. However, for externally caused scars, the readings offer an external remedy: camphorated oil. At the time this reading was given the oil available was camphorated olive oil. Today camphorated cottonseed oil is the only type sold.

Q-4. Are the scars on the legs or stomach detrimental in any way to the proper functioning of the body?
A-4. Little or no hindrance. These may be aided in being removed by sufficient time, precaution and persistence in activity; by the massage over those portions of small quantities at a time of tincture of myrrh and olive oil, and camphorated oil. These would be massaged at different times, to be sure; one one day and the other the second day from same—see? In preparing the olive oil and tincture of myrrh, heat the oil and add the myrrh—equal portions, only preparing such a quantity as would be used at each application. The camphorated oil may be obtained in quantity. Only massage such quantities as the cuticle and epidermis will absorb. This will require, to be sure, a long period, but remember the whole surface may be entirely changed if this is done persistently and consistently. In the massaging, do not massage so roughly as to produce irritation. The properties are to be absorbed. Do not merely pat the solution on, and do not use tufts of cotton or other properties to dab it on—dip the fingertips into the

solution, and it won't hurt the fingers either—it'll be good for them! and massage into affected portions.

Q-5. Would an electrical instrument be of assistance in removing the scars?

A-5. There are those instruments that may be helpful, but it would require their use in the hands of experienced individuals—and then the results would not be as effectual or as well done as nature's methods in applying properties such as outlined. For, the therapeutic value of the properties given to the skin itself is as follows: As given, as known and held by the ancients more than the present modes of medication, olive oil—properly prepared (hence pure olive oil should always be used)—is one of the most effective agents for stimulating muscular activity, or mucous-membrane activity, that may be applied to a body. Olive oil, then combined with the tincture of myrrh will be very effective; for the tincture of myrrh acts with the pores of the skin in such a manner as to strike in, causing the circulation to be carried to affected parts where tissue has been in the nature of folds—or scar tissue, produced from superficial activity from the active forces in the body itself, in making for coagulation in any portion of the system, whether external or internal. And, as indicated in the specific conditions referred to in relation to this body, will be *most* effectual. The camphorated oil is merely the same basic force (olive oil) to which has been added properties of camphor in more or less its raw or original state, than the spirits of same. Such activity in the epidermis is not only to produce soothing to affected areas but to stimulate the circulation in such effectual ways and manners as to combine with the other properties in bringing what will be determined, in the course of two to two and a half years, a new skin!   440-3

This concludes a broad survey of Cayce's theory of skin problems. These concepts differ in many respects from current popular ideas about these problems, but after studying them carefully their basis in common sense becomes apparent.

For more information relating to this article, see the following items in the Individual Reference File: Diet; Eliminations; Eliminants; Complexion; Drugless Therapy; and the *Circulating Files* (available to A.R.E. members) on Athlete's Foot; Castor Oil Packs; Complexion: Cosmetics; Indigestion and Gastritis; and Scars.

PSORIASIS—
HOPE FOR THE AFFLICTED

by John O.A. Pagano, D.C.

What Is Psoriasis?

When one embarks on a study of psoriasis, he will soon discover that there is no dearth of material. Literally, volumes have been written on the subject throughout the years. Some students believe that there are references to this particular disease even in Biblical writings.

Psoriasis has been described as a fairly common skin disease (six to eight million victims in America alone with 150,000 new cases each year); it is characterized by thickened, reddish patches of skin covered with heavy whitish scales. Although not painful (in most cases), the scaly sores may be disfiguring and a source of mental anguish. Elbows, knees, lower back, and scalp are the most commonly affected areas, although psoriasis can develop anywhere and everywhere on the skin, including the nails.

The victims of psoriasis often suffer a great deal of social discrimination. Because of the disease's appearance, employers and fellow workers are reluctant to hire or work with a psoriatic due to a mistaken idea that the disease is contagious. Psoriasis is not a contagious disease and cannot be caught from or given to others. Although, in some cases, there does seem to be a tendency for it to occur in families, there are just as many, if not more, cases in which it has never cropped up in other members of a family.

From the standpoint of orthodox medicine, the "cause" of psoriasis still remains a mystery. Government responsibility for psoriasis research lies largely with the National Institute of Arthritis, Metabolism, and Digestive Diseases in Bethesda, Maryland. The researchers know what happens to the surface cells in psoriasis, but the cause still eludes them.

At present, medical science offers three major topical (external) treatments: (1) crude coal tar ointments, (2) anthralin pastes (both often used with ultraviolet light), and (3) corticosteroid creams.

The latest concept, being used experimentally at Columbia Presbyterian Medical Center in New York, is a drug (methoxsalen) taken by mouth. The patient is subsequently exposed to ultraviolet light of a special longwave length. This process, "photochemotherapy," is not a permanent cure for psoriasis, although it appears to clear the skin lesions. Doctors are not sure of the side effects of such treatments, since it is only in the investigative stage.

The aforementioned methods may offer temporary relief, to be sure, but I dare say they are doomed to eventual failure for the simple reason that researchers are not looking in the right place for the cause of psoriasis! Looking to the skin for the cause of psoriasis is like looking to the lower leg for the cause of sciatica. As chiropractors, we are trained to seek out the origin of the nerve root (in the case of sciatica, of course, this being the 3-4-5L and S1 and 2 spinal segments).

I had yet to find an article on psoriasis that seemed to go beyond the surface of the skin in attempting to find the cause and treatment for this unwanted disease; that is, until I came upon the works of Edgar Cayce. Here, for the first time, an answer was given—not to be accepted simply at face value, but to be tried, tested and evaluated.

Here was a man whose primary desire throughout his life was to be an aid to suffering humanity. Not trained in the healing sciences (he was a photographer), he was able to place himself in a trance at will and when asked specific questions by those around him, including doctors and scientists, would give answers to various problems (particularly on health) that, when followed through, invariably brought forth curative results.

What did this man named Edgar Cayce, with such an amazing ability to tap unknown sources of information, have to say about psoriasis? Let's find out.

The Cause of Psoriasis

According to the Cayce readings, the external skin lesions are a manifestation of an *internal* disorder—namely, a thinning of the walls of the intestinal tract causing a "seepage" of toxins through these walls into the circulation and lymphatics. To quote directly from a reading for a 74-year-old woman:

There are disturbing conditions which prevent the better physical functioning in this body. These have to do primarily with an intestinal disorder and the lack of proper coordination in the eliminating systems. There are those conditions, then, in the duodenum and through the jejunum where there are the effects as if there were tiny thinned walls, as if the walls of the duodenum had been smoothed, rather than the folds that should exist with the gastric flow which should come through these areas at the periods of digestions. The results are a disturbance in the blood supply and an irritation in the superficial circulation, so that those areas in the epidermis show eliminations that should be carried through alimentary canal, for these are being eliminated through perspiratory system.   3373-1

The logical course of action to take, therefore, would be primarily to detoxify the body and maintain this condition after the process has been accomplished. This may be achieved by the following: (1) colonic irrigations; (2) strict dietary control; (3) specific herbal drinks; (4) adjustments of the spine; and (5) as a topical measure, external applications. To be more specific about each measure, described by Edgar Cayce, we present the following.

The high colonic irrigation:
The first measure to aid in relieving the body of accumulated toxins is the high colonic irrigation. This should be administered professionally.
A colonic is given at the start of treatment. Seven days later another is administered and two weeks later another. After a period of at least one month or six weeks, a fourth colonic may be given.

Proper diet for the psoriasis patient:
The diet should be aimed at promoting alkalinity in the body, thus bringing about a better acid-base balance to the entire system. (See the acid-alkaline food chart on page 126.)
The following must be adhered to:
1. Eat many fresh fruits and vegetables. One meal a day, usually lunch, should consist of raw vegetables only. You may use oil or salad dressing—no vinegar!
2. Cooked vegetables with no meat, other than fish, fowl and lamb, may be taken. Eat a good quantity of seafood.
3. Eliminate fats, sweets and pastries!

4. Have at least three vegetables that grow above the ground for each one that grows below the ground.

5. Wine is permissable in moderation, but no other liquor.

6. Eat large quantities of *lettuce* as well as celery, watercress, and similar foods (unless the roughage causes irritation to an underlying ulcer or a colitis condition). Lettuce is a blood purifier!

7. Keep away from red meats, ham and rare or roasted steak. Completely avoid fried foods.

Note: A general guide showing the relative acid-base balance of various foods is included with this article. The psoriasis patient should basically avoid those foods listed as acid-forming foods (with the exception of fish, fowl and lamb) and stress those foods listed as alkaline-forming foods (with the exception of tomatoes).

At least three mornings each week we would have the rolled or crushed or cracked whole wheat, that is not cooked too long so as to destroy the whole vitamin force in same, but this will add to the body the proper proportions of iron, silicon and the vitamins necessary to build up the blood supply that makes for resistance in the system. We at other periods would have citrus fruits, citrus fruit juices, the yolk of eggs (preferably soft boiled or coddled—not the white portions of same), browned bread with butter, Ovaltine or milk, or coffee, provided there is no milk or cream put in same. Occasionally stewed fruits, as baked apples with cream, stewed figs, stewed raisins, stewed prunes or stewed apricots—these may be taken in preference to same. But do not eat citrus fruits at the same meal with cereals or gruels or any of the breakfast foods.

During the morning we would have a malted milk, between this and the lunch hour, you see; preferably with a raw egg in same, or there may be a taste or two of the spirits frumenti—only sufficient to make for strengthening.

Noons—preferably raw fresh vegetables; none cooked at this meal. These would consist of tomatoes [see Note #1 of *Basic Foods* chart], lettuce, celery, spinach, carrots, beet tops, mustard, onions or the like (not cucumbers) that make for the purifying of the *humor* in the lymph blood as this is absorbed by the lacteal ducts as it is digested. We would not take any quantities of soups or broths at this period.

Evenings—broths or soups may be taken in a small measure at this meal; but let it consist principally of vegetables that are well-cooked and a little of the meats such as lamb, fish, fowl—these are preferable. No fried foods for the body.   840-1

Herbal drinks and external applications:

1. The primary herbs for the correction of psoriasis are the American Yellow Saffron tea, Slippery Elm Bark Powder, Camomile tea, and Mullein tea. The Yellow Saffron tea should be taken more often than the others and alternated with the Camomile tea.

2. External applications consist primarily of baths using Cuticura soap, followed by Cuticura ointment, then an application of Resinol ointment gently rubbed into the lesions. Sleep with it on overnight, bathing in the morning again with Cuticura soap.

3. Massage the body periodically with a mixture of equal parts of olive oil and peanut oil. After the massage, if conditions permit, bathe in sunlight—but not to the point of becoming sunburned. If exposure to direct sunlight is not possible, the *proper* use of ultraviolet light may be very helpful, but extreme caution must be applied here. One should not expose any one area of the body to ultraviolet light for over a period of 1 to 1½ minutes. Be sure you have eye protectors and that the light is at a distance of at least 40 inches.

4. It has been found very helpful to apply warm castor oil on major circumscribed lesions, then wrap the area with Saran wrap, and leave it that way for several hours. This will help heal the surface cells. Repeat this method at least twice a week until the area clears up. The olive oil/peanut oil mixture may also be used in this method. As part of the external applications, Epsom salts baths may be added as home therapy. Instructions follow.

Epsom salts bath:

Epsom salts baths have proved to be extremely helpful in removing psoriasis lesions. However, if there are open sores, such as cracked heels or feet, the burning sensation is usually too much to bear and it is recommended to wait until these inner layers of skin are healed before taking the baths.

Directions: Saturate 4 pounds of Epsom salts in a bathtub. Fill the tub ¾ full with comfortably hot water (a temperature of about 102-104 degrees). Be sure to stir the salts thoroughly. Immerse yourself in the tub, but as the water cools, gradually add hot water so it is always comfortably hot. Then soak for 20 minutes. One should take these baths twice a week, then shower down and use the Cuticura soap.

Caution: (1) Do not take Epsom salts baths if you have a heart

Basic Foods to Eat or Avoid for the Psoriasis Patient

Eat large quantities of the following:

Avoid the following foods—except fish, fowl and lamb (never fried):

Alkaline-Forming Foods

apples	grapefruit	peaches
apricots	honey	pears
berries	lemons	pineapples
dates	limes	raisins
figs (unsulphured)	oranges	small prunes

All vegetables—fresh and dehydrated, *except* legumes (dried peas, beans, and lentils) and rhubarb.

asparagus	green peas	radishes
beets	kohlrabi	rutabaga
cabbage	lettuce	spinach
carob	mushrooms	sprouts
carrots	olives (ripe)	string beans
cauliflower	onions	sweet potatoes*
celery	oyster plant	tomatoes*
eggplant	parsnips	turnips

Milk—all forms: buttermilk, clabber, sour milk, cottage cheese, cheese.

Acid-Forming Foods

Animal fats and vegetable oils—large prunes, plums, cranberries, rhubarb.

All cereal grains—and other such products, as bread, breakfast foods, rolled oats, corn flakes, corn meal mush, polished rice, etc. (Brown rice is less acid-forming.)

All high starch and protein foods—white sugar, syrups made from white sugar. (Starchy foods in combination with fruits or proteins are acid combinations and should be avoided.)

Nuts—peanuts, English walnuts, pecans, filberts, coconut.

Legumes—dried beans, dried peas, lentils.

Meats—beef, pork, lamb, veal.

Poultry—chicken, turkey, duck, goose, guinea hen, game.

Visceral meats—heart, brains, kidney, liver, sweetbreads, thymus.

Egg whites. (Yolks are not acid-forming.)

Note: *1. Tomatoes (including tomato sauces) seem to have an adverse effect on psoriasis; therefore, they are to be avoided.
2. Drink 6 to 8 glasses of water daily.
3. Do not combine cereal with citrus fruits or juices. When combined, they are acidic.
4. At least one meal (usually lunch) should consist of raw vegetables only.

problem or high blood pressure. (2) When taking hot baths of any kind, be sure to have someone nearby in case you faint or are overcome by dizziness.

Using Saffron tea and Slippery Elm Powder:
Saffron tea: Place a pinch of the Yellow Saffron tea in a cup of boiling water and allow it to stand for 30 minutes; then strain it, and drink it each evening when ready to retire.

Saffron tea was described in the readings as a cleanser for the kidneys and liver as well as an aid in healing the inner walls of the intestinal tract.

Ground Elm Bark: Occasionally, about two or three times a week, drink Elm water. This is made by taking a pinch of Ground Elm (between your thumb and forefinger) and putting it in a cup filled with *warm,* not boiling, water; let it stand 30 minutes. Drink this preferably in the morning rather than when the Saffron tea would be taken. If you find this difficult to take, the readings suggest adding ice to the drink.

Adjustments of the spine:
Spinal adjustments (chiropractic or osteopathic) are recommended throughout the readings as a major health measure to prevent many forms of illness, and psoriasis is no exception. However, one reading even describes a certain subluxation (misaligned vertebra) as a possible cause of psoriasis.

Certain spinal segments to be adjusted were specifically recommended, with special attention being placed at the level of the 6th and 7th dorsal vertebrae. As stated by Cayce:

... we find that there are pressures also existing in the areas of the 6th, 7th dorsal that upset the coordination of circulation through the kidneys and the liver ...

Then, in making applications for corrections here we would first through osteopathic adjustments correct those subluxations upon the right side at the 6th and 7th dorsal and then coordinate the 3rd cervical, the 9th dorsal and through the lumbar, with such corrections. There should only be required about twelve adjustments, if properly made, coordinating the muscular forces in areas where the sympathetic and cerebrospinal systems coordinate in the greater measure. 5016-1

The entire principle in treating the psoriasis patient is to

Adjustments of the Spine:

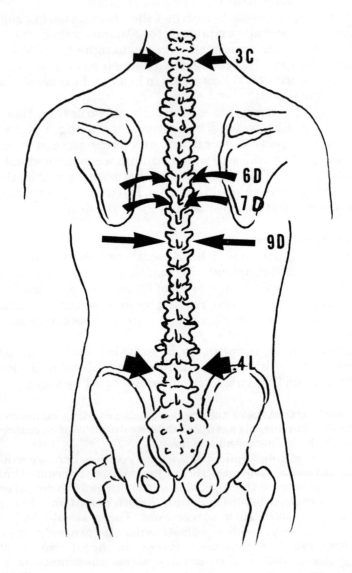

For psoriasis, adjust the areas of the 6th and 7th dorsal; "then coordinate the 3rd cervical, the 9th dorsal and through the lumbar. . . " (5016-1)

clear the blood and lymphatics of accumulated toxins and prevent further pollution.

A 28-year-old woman asked the question, "Is there an absolute cure for psoriasis?" The sleeping Cayce answered:

Most of this is found in diet. There is a cure. It requires patience, persistence—and right thinking also.   2455-2

On Right Thinking

It is an established fact not only in the readings but in modern science, that the attitude of the patient (and doctor!) is as important, or more important, than the therapy itself. A belief that you will be healed increases your chances of success to an invaluable degree.

The body expects to be in distress and it remains in distress. For what one builds in the subconscious of itself, it becomes— rather as a habit, like any form of activity by the voluntary motions of the body-forces.   3287-2

Therefore, a right mental attitude means expecting good to come to you. One reading tells us: ". . . truly, he that expects little will not be disappointed" (505-1), while another states, ". . . he that expects much—if he lives and uses that in hand day by day—shall be full to running over." (557-3)

Many fixations are so deeply rooted in our subconscious minds that the cause of the disease often evades us. To illustrate: An interesting case brought to my attention was that of a young girl who was completely cured of psoriasis, only to have it return on the Mother's Day following the death of her mother. The patient herself provided an explanation.

She, as a child, was afflicted with psoriasis, and her devoted mother gave her more love and attention than the rest of her children to offset the heartbreak of this disease. The psoriasis did in time clear up. (I am not aware of the course of treatment followed.) However, the disease returned phenomenally all over her body on Mother's Day after her mother had died! It then cleared up again as the holiday passed.

To the author, the above case does not indicate a return of toxicity to the body, but it demonstrates the incredible powers of the subconscious faculty within each and every one of us.

Therefore, patients with psoriasis should guard and select the thoughts that enter their minds as carefully as they would choose the right food intake, if success is to be realized.

From the readings the following may be formulated:

1. Spinal adjustments aid in getting to one root cause of psoriasis; namely, incoordination of the eliminating system and diminished proper circulation to the intestines, causing a breakdown of the intestinal walls. Both systems are controlled by the nerves, particularly in the areas of the 6-7D and balancing of 3C-9D and 4L.

2. Saffron tea and Slippery Elm heal the plaques and lining of the intestinal walls, helping to prevent further seepage of toxins through the walls. The Saffron also cleanses the kidneys and liver.

3. The diet prevents further build-up of toxins by ingesting foods that are more "pure" in nature and are natural eliminants.

4. The oils (peanut/olive oil mixture and castor oil applications) heal the surface cells of the skin. This condition is also aided by Cuticura soap and ointment.

5. The colonics remove toxins that have accumulated for years in the large intestine, thus aiding the therapy's basic principle—internal purification of the body.

The photographic evidence, included here, of successfully treated cases of psoriasis does not particularly serve as "proof" that all cases will respond as favorably in such a short time (although they may in most cases). More time and similar results are necessary to form definite conclusions. These photographs, taken by the author, show what happened in these particular cases.

There have been unsuccessful cases to date. However, in every case, the patient expected results too soon, did not follow instructions, was discouraged by others, or had a poor doctor-patient relationship—in other words, "bad vibes"!

The following photographs have been reproduced with written consent of the patient or his guardian. (See pp. 133-139.)

The Question of Recurrence

To relieve a patient of a problem is one thing. To prevent the problem from recurring is quite another and, of course, the more desirable. Any serious researcher must consider the question of recurrence if the work is to have lasting significance.

Since this form of therapy for treating psoriasis is just beginning to gather successful results, it is somewhat premature to offer definite statements. However, in regard to the cases herein depicted, the following facts are offered:

1. In the case of William Culmone: His lesions cleared up within a three-month period and have not returned after a period of one-and-a-half years.

2. In the case of young Andrew Senzon: He was virtually clear in a period of three months and continues to remain clear. No significant period of time has lapsed to observe recurrence.

3. In the case of Barbara Kowalski: The disease cleared in about a four-month period. There was a slight recurrence when she went off her diet, but it was quickly brought under control. Now, three months after clearing, there is no recurrence.

From a common-sense point of view, it seems reasonable to assume that the patient must stay on the diet and carry out periodically some of the measures for a period of six months to a year after all lesions have cleared. If, after this period, there is a recurrence when the patient goes off the diet, one must then adopt these dietary measures as a way of life—a small price to pay considering the alternative.

Note: The author recognizes the fact that not all measures suggested in the readings are mentioned in this article; for example, such treatments as fume baths, wet-cell appliance, the hand-held violet ray, and the mixture of sulphur, cream of tartar and Rochelle salts as an eliminant. These measures, of course, are recommended—provided they comply with the physician's state regulations. From a practical point of view, however, the treatments presented here have proved to be sufficient to bring about within a three-month period remarkable results in most cases.

Final Comments

With the world desperately craving a better way of life—which we somehow know inwardly is our birthright—is it any wonder that people are more and more seeking answers that according to "accepted" procedures may be considered unorthodox? Let us not forget that at one time books were considered works of the devil; tomatoes, poisonous; and innocent citizens labeled "witches" were burned at the stake. (A study from the *New York Times,* March 31, 1976, indicates that these people may simply have been victims of eating contaminated bread which caused the hallucinations.) Can you not remember when chiropractic was considered an unscientific cult?

The psychic readings of Edgar Cayce offer a new dimension in thinking. (One of them stresses that "more research" is needed.) Although they are not as yet "accepted" with the stamp of officialdom, does this mean that the information obtained is invalid? The difference is that these readings offer a definite procedure to follow with no apparent harm to the patient. In the 8,976 health readings, each patient receiving the reading obtained satisfacory results in practically every case, *if the recommendations were followed faithfully!* Case after case was cured (yes, cured!) of the ailment when all else failed. Is there hope for the victims of multiple sclerosis, muscular dystrophy, or arthritis? According to the Cayce readings, there certainly is! There are numerous files of readings advising what may be done, stressing the cause as well as the procedure to follow.

We are here on this earth for basically one profound reason— to *enjoy living!* Good health is essential to that principle. We are not meant to struggle for life; we are meant to live our lives to the fullest. If we come short of that purpose, it is because we have violated some principle of successful living, either on purpose or through ignorance.

Only through knowledge can we overcome ignorance. Knowledge (or truth) may be obtained by painstaking research, handed down from generation to generation, or—as is increasingly being recognized—by direct subconscious communication with what Carl Jung calls the "collective unconscious." Whatever the method of obtaining information, what difference does it make if the truth is realized?

Further research into the Edgar Cayce readings by interested medical doctors, chiropractors, and osteopaths offers a new spring of hope in the relief of man's ills. It will prove, as Walt Whitman stated so aptly, "that man is not all contained between his hat and his boots."

See "References" on p. 140.

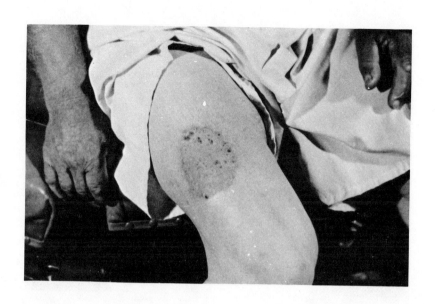

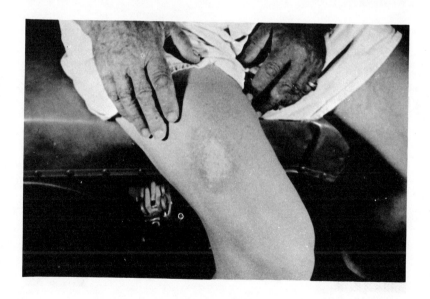

Patient: William Culmone Age: 65 years Afflicted: 15 years
Top photo taken 7/25/75 at start of treatment.
Bottom photo taken 10/16/75.

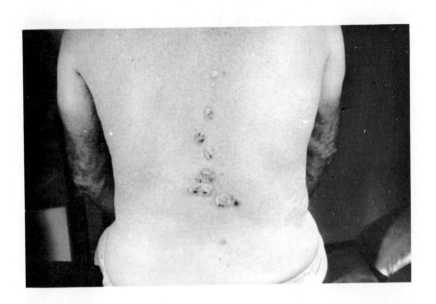

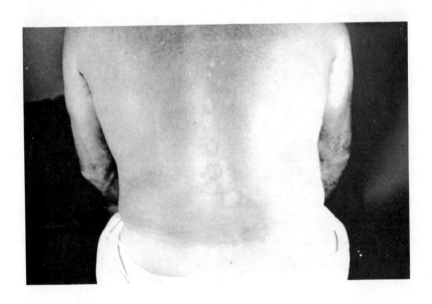

Patient: William Culmone
Top photo taken 7/25/75 at start of treatment.
Bottom photo taken 10/16/75.

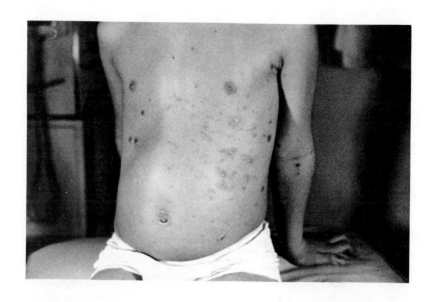

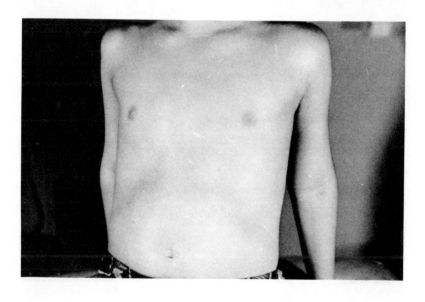

Patient: Andrew Senzon Age: 5 years Afflicted: 4 years
Top photo taken 1/13/77. Treatment started 12/17/76.
Bottom photo taken 4/5/77—less than four months from start of treatment.

135

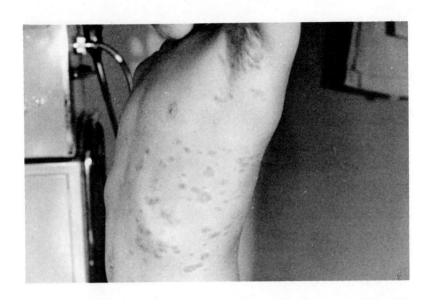

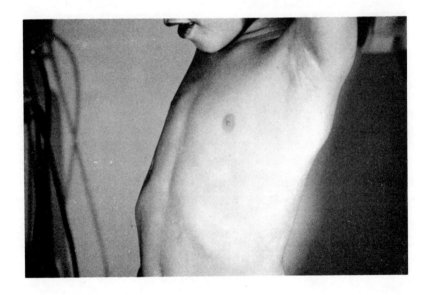

Patient: Andrew Senzon
Top photo taken 1/13/77. Treatment started 12/17/76.
Bottom photo taken 4/5/77—less than four months from start of treatment.

136

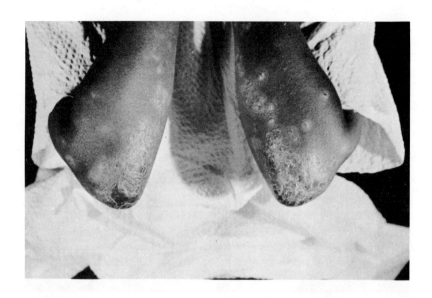

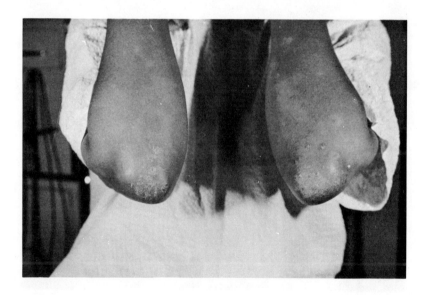

Patient: Barbara Kowalski Age: 32 years Afflicted: 2 years
Top photo taken 9/3/76 at start of treatment.
Bottom photo taken 3/10/77. Patient was clear by 1/3/77.

137

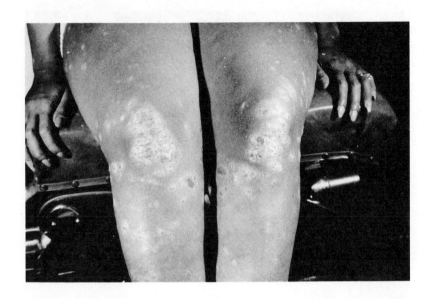

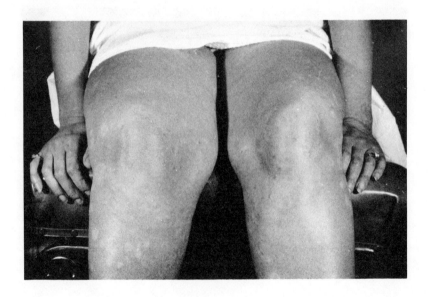

Patient: Barbara Kowalski
Top photo taken 9/3/76 at start of treatment.
Bottom photo taken 1/3/77—four months from start of treatment.

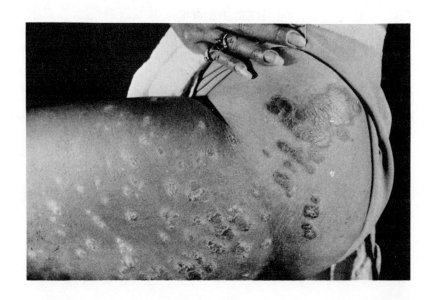

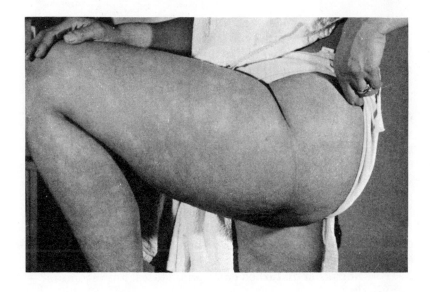

Patient: Barbara Kowalski
Top photo taken 9/3/76 at start of treatment.
Bottom photo taken 3/10/77. Patient was clear by 1/3/77.

REFERENCES

1. Circulating Files. Vols. 1 & 2 on *Psoriasis*. A.R.E. Press: Virginia Beach, Va.

2. *HEW—Fact Sheet on Psoriasis*. U.S. Department of Health, Education & Welfare, February, 1976.

3. Knox, Gerald M. "How to Cope with Psoriasis." *Better Homes and Gardens,* October, 1975, p. 44.

4. Lansford, Frederick D., Jr., M.D. *Physician's Reference Notebook*. William A. McGarey, M.D., ed. A.R.E. Press: Virginia Beach, Va., 1968, pp. 188-195.

5. North, Carolyn, R.N., and Gerald D. Weinstein, M.D. "Treatment of Psoriasis." *American Journal of Nursing,* 1976, pp. 410-412.

6. Reilly, Harold J., D.Ph.T., D.S., and Ruth Hagy Brod. *The Edgar Cayce Handbook for Health Through Drugless Therapy*. New York: Macmillan, 1975, pp. 55-58.

7. Stearn, Jess. *Edgar Cayce, the Sleeping Prophet*. New York: Doubleday & Co., Inc., 1967.

8. Troward, Thomas. *The Edinburgh Lectures on Mental Science*. Dodd-Mead Books, 1909.

Musical Medication

Music therapy is gaining in this country as well as in Europe. Emotions are certainly quieted down or aroused by a variety of musical compositions. Much has been written about this, and we are all familiar with the manner in which one type of music soothes us to sleep while another stirs our martial instincts. A clipping sent to me tells of music and its use in Europe. The works of the masters are being played through a device, developed by a Frenchman, that influences cell tissue by transforming sounds into direct vibrations. The patient listens while the tunes are further relayed through electrodes attached to the body.

A physician in Rome has been using Bach fugues to treat indigestion, and it has been found that Mozart is an ideal choice when working with rheumatism. Beethoven is considered good for hernias, while Handel helps "broken hearts" and other disturbed emotional states. For insomnia?— Schubert.

While part of the effect reported might be psychological, it might also be induced through the sense of hearing. Yet the answer may lie in the vibratory influence brought to the body directly.

CYSTITIS—MANIFESTATION OF A PHYSIOLOGICAL IMBALANCE

by Fred D. Lansford, Jr., M.D.

Presented to the Third Annual Symposium of the Medical Research Division of the Edgar Cayce Foundation in Phoenix, Arizona, on January 12, 1970.

Textbooks list the causes of cystitis as many and varied. In fact, the causes and specific areas of distress are such that it is often preferable to refer to an infection in this area as a urinary tract infection, rather than an inflammation of a specific anatomical site, such as urethritis, cystitis, trigonitis, and so forth. This terminology may have been brought about by the realization that while the symptoms may be localized to a certain area, the disease process usually involves several structures within the urinary tract.

The prevalance of urinary tract infection is said to be around thirty times more prevalent in women than in men. This is thought to be due to the shortened urethra or the closer proximity of the bladder to the external urethral orifice in women than in men. According to this theory, bladder pathogens, or bacteria, invade the bladder via the shortened urethra and, by their ability to collect in greater numbers in the female bladder, set up an infection.

Stasis of the urine also tends to play a major contributing part in the formation of inflammation or infection in the bladder itself. Due to the structure of the female pelvis, especially following the childbearing process, residual urine is likely to remain. Urine is good culture medium and, on a mixed diet, is slightly acid. The pH is about 6. This is due to the end products of metabolism which give several acids of oxidation and carbonic acid or the bicarbonate salt, the biphosphate and the sulfate. The food of herbivorous animals, on the contrary, gives many basic end products. The salts of tartaric, mallic, citric acids when oxidized, set free a fixed base, such as sodium or potassium. Because of this, the urine of herbivora is alkaline and, in people on a vegetarian diet, also becomes alkaline.

The extreme values of urinary pH are about from 4.8 to 8.2. When the pH of the urine reaches 7 or greater, that is, slightly alkaline, a suspicion of infection is considered.

The intestinal organisms, especially *E. coli,* are the most frequent of all bacteria found in the urinary tract. These are thought to cause a major portion of cystitis due to the frequent association with the inflammatory process. I have no reason, really, to doubt that this is true. However, it is too often assumed that the mere presence of bacteria causes infection, and we fail to recall that it takes a rather overwhelming number of organisms in order to bring about infection in an otherwise healthy urinary tract.

Certain studies have been done on this in which *E. coli* have been injected into the urinary tract of healthy male subjects in rather large numbers without causing infection. Yet, when the same number of *E. coli* organisms are injected into the urinary tracts where a neurological deficit exists, such as paralysis from a stroke or from spinal trauma, then an infection can take place. This• has caused me to wonder if the urinary tract infections that we so often treat in our clinical experience are not really the result of a large number of bacteria being present that somehow find their way into the bladder, but are actually the result of disease process rather than the cause of it.

What would this disease process be? If this is true, it might be that most of the bacteria we find in the urine during a bout of cystitis are the result of a secondary infection, secondary to some devitalizing process within the system that has caused either a stasis of urine flow or has so interfered with the normal physiology or physiological processes on a cellular level as to render them unable to resist the few bacteria normally present. Bladder infection, then, might be more the result of a loss of cellular vitality within the urinary tract, rather than the sudden, often unexplained presence of a large number of bacteria or other virulent organisms appearing in the bladder.

When I began working on the Circulating File on cystitis, I reviewed some fifty readings to try to get some of Cayce's ideas on the subject. Then I began to try to read through his manner of speaking to find what he was really trying to say. This was perhaps the most difficult aspect because there were certain things that I did not understand, certain anatomical terminology that I did not grasp. I had to dig through, formulate ideas and see if these ideas worked. If they did not, then I had to toss them aside and start over.

Eighteen cases were used to illustrate the importance of what Cayce said. Of these eighteen cases, fourteen were females and four were males. The ages ran from 31 years to 65 years. In looking at some of the causes of cystitis, as found by Edgar Cayce in these eighteen people, since some had more than one cause listed, it was not just organisms present in the urinary tract that caused the conditions. This was the interesting thing. As to exactly what it was, I was not sure, even after I read and sometimes re-read these readings. What was he getting *at?* What was he speaking *of?*

I came up with these ideas. An overacid condition was present in four cases as one of the chief causes. Exactly what was meant by an overacid condition, I was not entirely sure. This is an area to investigate further because there are many causes or many different things that can contribute to an overacid condition—infection, trauma or diet. Fear, anger, the most retarding emotions can also produce an overacid condition in the body. Maybe we are talking about trauma on another level here when we speak of these more emotional aspects.

There were three blood circulatory problems. Two were anemias, and one was merely referred to as an improper circulation. There were four spinal "lesions." These ranged in area from T-6 to the coccyx with two of them at the level of T-9. Multiple pelvic adhesions was one cause. Trauma at childbirth was another. Pelvic inflammation occurred in two cases, and a prolapsed segment of the colon with accumulated toxins absorbed in the system and eliminated through the kidneys was also causative in one case. The largest classification within the group were those causes related to the liver and the gall duct and the surrounding organs of digestion—what Cayce refers to as the hepatic circulation. This is a term which I thought I understood when I first started. The hepatic circulation—that's the liver circulation. It sounds easy, but as I read into this, I began to find that it was not easy. It did not quite fit. At least it was not the hepatic circulation as I had learned, or thought I had learned, in medical school.

Of the eighteen individuals of these readings, fifteen had

difficulties or imbalances in the hepatic circulation. These abnormalities of the hepatic circulation ranged all the way from cirrhosis, resulting from prolonged ether inhalation by a nurse-anesthetist, to such vague causes as torpidity of the liver and incoordination between liver and kidneys.

Now, Cayce mentions a polarity between the liver and the kidneys in the body.

Then there is that circulation called the hepatic, as indicated, wherein there is the *coordinant* reaction between the liver *and* the kidneys. The liver is an excretory as well as a secretive organ. The kidneys are *secretive* and take *from* the system, also from the liver and from the general circulation of the whole abdominal area, poisons that are not eliminated through other ways and manners.

When toxic forces arise in the body from the inflammation through the abdominal area, or through the uterus itself [this was a case of pelvic inflammation], combined with the disturbances through lack of proper elimination in the alimentary canal, *then* we have a sparse activity of the bladder or of the kidneys through the bladder. Then this produces in the body an irritation, owing to the great excess of acidity, that produces a burning even through the clitoris and the mouth of the uterus and in the portions of the body.

This is not an indication that the kidneys are involved but that the activity of the whole hepatic circulation and the organs or eliminations through these portions of the system become involved in same.   1140-2

This was a challenge. This told me that I was getting into some factors here with which I was not familiar. I noticed as I read through the readings and as he kept referring to this hepatic circulation, that I was getting more confused than enlightened. This was only because of preconceived ideas I had as to what was meant. It shook me up a little bit and made me dig even deeper.

Then, he made mention of the upper hepatic circulation, as well as the lower hepatic circulation. His use of these terms did not fit with the arterial and the portal circulatory systems of the liver, as I had at first assumed. To make the matter even more involved, he kept referring to the kidneys as a part of the lower hepatic circulation, and, in my mind's eye, I just could not quite trace any part of the portal circulation to the kidneys. After much head scratching and re-reading of this material, I concluded that what Cayce was referring to as the upper hepatic circulation was the stomach, the duodenum, the pancreas, the spleen, the liver, and the gall bladder. The remainder of the portal circulation that is through perhaps the lower part of the small intestine and the large bowel and together with the drainage from the kidneys, he was calling the lower hepatic circulation. It was then that I was able to get the gist of what Cayce was saying about the underlying causes of cystitis.

It might be a good idea here to quote again from Cayce and give you what he had to say directly. This is one of the things that confused me, and I must admit it still, in part, confuses me a little. He said:

As an organ (for the more perfect understanding of the body, for this may be disputed by some), the liver and kidneys form the hepatic circulation. The blood supply of the whole body goes through the liver twice, even to once through the heart.

1140-2

Perhaps Cayce meant by that last statement that it goes through the liver by two different routes, rather than twice. Whether this is correct or not, it seems a possible interpretation.

Another case has this to say:

We have at times the condition with the lower portion of the hepatic circulation; when the kidneys are affected, not other than sympathetically, in their attempt to aid in the elimination of these toxic forces that are created in the body. A burning through the urethra, with the evacuation of the bladder, occurs at times.

These are from a form of acidity.

2462-1

Here we see the kidneys attempting to compensate for imbalances in other areas of the body. In this particular instance, the trouble was with lesions of the spine, which, among other things, brought about a delayed emptying of the duodenum and began to upset the digestive system.

Cayce frequently referred to the acid condition of the body. This is one of the characteristics present in a cold or upper respiratory infection. He alluded to certain aspects of the diet as contributing to this overacid condition—such foods as sweets, starches, pastries, and the like. He frequently advised fresh fruits, vegetables, the more alkaline foods, as a means of correcting the system.

He often referred to the sympathetic action or reflex action of the urinary tract when he linked it to diseased organs elsewhere in the body:

That pressure in its impulse to the liver prevents the proper assimilation; thus unbalancing the chemical reactions to that assimilating; causing periods of a fullness in the pit of the stomach, or non-activity of that area of the duodenum emptying into the lacteals with the secretions from liver (or gall duct), spleen and pancreas.

Thus we have at times, from this condition, an irregular or reflex activity to the kidneys; causing a scant but oft activity of the bladder at periods—at others a *lack* of activity, and the producing of a burning or a high sensitiveness in the act of passing the urine through the urethra.

Neither of these, as first indicated, is organic in itself...

2402-1

This is important—purely reflex and functional impulses based upon a deflection from a highly sensitive body and attempts of a good physical body to take care of or to meet these excesses in the system. He is saying something here that just did not quite go along with what I learned in medical school. I *think* it is something that perhaps I might have needed to learn, to understand exactly what cystitis amounts to—its pathology in a chronic case or maybe even in an acute case, where there is inflammation perhaps in other organs and the intestinal tract, rather than merely in the bladder itself. Rather than just treating the bladder with certain drugs, we might need to look into the entire organism, get back to treating the entire person, rather than a set of organs or one organ in particular.

In another case Cayce refers to what is apparently a sympathetic reflex action in the body, and indicates that, if some other part of the system becomes diseased and impaired or insulted, then through the autonomic nervous system, this impairment can also cause a reflex action to take place within the kidneys or the bladder. Perhaps a spasm of the blood supply and the irritation from the acid might tend to cause inflammation of the epithelial cells, causing a congestion and a stasis of the lymph flow, preventing the removal of certain waste products which would add to the condition in and around the bladder and causing a build-up over a period of time. We could treat, then, the organisms that might begin to be present in larger numbers in the bladder as a result of all this process, but this would be merely getting rid of some of the organisms, not only in the bladder, but also in the intestinal tract where *E. coli* plays a vital role. It would get rid of some of these other organisms in the body that maybe the body needs. Maybe it did have a little too much in the bladder, and we might be assuming this was causing it. It might even be causing a little bit of inflammation in the bladder as a result of an inflammation that was already present, but that might not really be the cause of it. It might be something else. What Cayce seems to be saying is that we would have to look, then, for reflex actions from other parts of the body.

Reading 2729-2 was given for a 38-year-old woman who had anemia and cirrhosis due to toxic anesthesia. She was a nurse-anesthetist who gave ether quite a bit, and, in doing so, she breathed the ether. Cayce said this was causing a whitish scarring of the liver, which we assume was cirrhosis:

> In the action of the digestion itself, these then function under strain, and the character of the excretions from the system at times indicate this, as does that effect as is produced upon the lower hepatic circulation, or the condition in the kidneys. The irritation at times for the bladder itself, though *not* an organic condition there—yet an irritation; rather as of a *burning*—produced by the attempt of the system to create an equilibrium in the full hepatic circulation . . .
> While the functioning of the organs as relate to the pelvis and the organs of those portions of the body suffer at times *under* these, these are rather reflexes.   2729-2

This is most interesting, for to treat a reflex with antibiotics can perhaps have some benefit, not to the reflex itself, but maybe to what is causing the reflex in other areas of the body.

He again mentions acidity in a reading for a person who had cholecystitis and cystitis, again a female, forty-two years of age.

Q-1. What causes the burning in the bladder? Can it be cured?
A-1. The irritations that arise from the super amount of acidity in the system. Using the douches as indicated, correcting the conditions in the upper hepatic circulation, we will find a great deal of help in these directions. This has not localized, and is constitutional.   1446-1

Another one on acidity: This person had lesions from the fifth dorsal to the ninth dorsal, and it caused a variable emptying of the duodenum into the lower part of the small intestine. This had produced some pathology in the liver and a toxic condition throughout the body. There were also some lesions in the coccygeal area which contributed to the overall imbalances in the system.

We have at times the condition with the lower portion of the hepatic circulation; when the kidneys are affected, not other than sympathetically, in their attempt to aid in the elimination of these toxic forces that are created in the body. A burning through the urethra, with the evacuation of the bladder, occurs at times.

These are from a form of acidity. This may produce such an effluvium in the blood as to cause at times an irritation in the superficial circulation; so that areas over the body will at times appear to be itchy, or as if there is a movement under the skin itself. 2462-1

In the way of poisons in the system, this is one where there was anemia, jejunal adhesions, and a form of strep in the body. He commented on other things that led me to believe that maybe he was referring to a state of regional ileitis when he said, "And these cause a great deal of disturbance at times through that area between the cecum and the upper portions of the jejunum." He said:

Adhesions and lesions in this area, then, are the basis or the causes of the greater disturbances.

These, acting upon the nerve reflex for the functioning of the liver and gall duct and the spleen and pancreas, have at times, brought those reflexes of a pressure in the greater blood supply itself . . .

These are only indications of the character or nature of the disturbances. These reflect at times, to be sure, upon the functioning between the upper and the lower hepatic circulation, causing a disturbance to the kidneys as they relate to the functioning through the activity of the bladder itself.

Hence those periods when the excess of this effluvium to be eliminated produces a burning sensation through the urethra at times in the eliminating of the poisons from the body itself. 2050-1

Now, in the hepatic circulation in a case of an adult female, he mentioned a hypertension tendency, irritations in the water she was ingesting, and fear, which he said played a part in the cause of her condition.

These causing certain forces, or bacilli to be thrown into the blood, which show the condition, especially as those through the hepatic circulation do; we find traces of this being acted upon and eliminated by the action of the excretory forces or functions of the liver itself, the effect being from the opposite pole of the kidneys, and the action of the hepatic circulation on these conditions—see?   3972-1

Cayce mentions the disturbed hepatic circulation in other readings, but *I think* this is enough to give you some idea that something is going on here, other than just in the bladder itself, and we have to find out what it is. I am not speaking of these cases where we do get a gross pyuria in the bladder and where, on cystoscopy, we find that there is infection and a lot of organisms present and where it is obvious that something needs to be done to eliminate the infection that is actually going on in the bladder. Sometimes that may involve antibiotics, but not just antibiotics. That may get rid of the bacteria. They may get rid of the pyuria temporarily or maybe even for several weeks or months, but until we can get at the initial underlying cause, we have not done a complete job. This may involve diet.

Cayce mentioned watermelon seed tea, which, incidentally does not taste too bad. It is a little unusual, and in my part of the country, where we have various herb doctors, when I start prescribing watermelon seed tea, some of my patients say, "Gee, I can get that over here across the mountain from old Mrs. So-and-so, who prescribes that." I have prescribed it anyway with varying results. Some people will take it. Some will not. Some will take it only until they get rid of the symptoms, without really having any insight into the fact that they need to cure more than just a set of symptoms that they have at the moment.

I have found in my practice that there are other causes of cystitis. A frequent cause of one acute stage of cystitis is a cold. Maybe not just a common cold, but one of these echo viruses, something like the enterocolic virus of the intestinal tract. In most colds, it has been my personal observation that there is an element (even though the symptoms are in the nose and the sinuses around in the throat, maybe in the lungs and upper respiratory tract) in the intestinal tract which is getting down into the hepatic circulation system, too. We have to, at least, be aware of this.

A cold does play a part, and flu plays an even bigger part because you can knock these flu viruses down but not out. They tend to come back recurrently in cycles, each time a little worse. This is why if you treat a urinary tract infection, it should be for a least a week and preferably two weeks with the usual set of drugs that we use, in order to make sure it is cured. I have noticed from personal observation, that you can treat it for two or three days and the symptoms will go away. They are not likely to come back if you treat the other part of the system, too. But if you are just treating the bladder, it may take two weeks for the other part of the system to correct itself enough to where it will not come back. I cannot say that this is the case always nor can I speak with authority on this. It is merely a theory that I entertain in my mind in treating this condition and in seeing it, wondering why some people get over it and other people do not, why we have chronic cases that do not seem to respond to anything and all of this.

This is an area that is open to further discussion and research in the readings. Maybe we can all learn more by reading and delving into the cause of the disease in the system itself.

I guess everybody has his own little bit of philosophy that he runs across in the readings that he feels he must give to the rest of us at times, and I have my own. This one in particular, I came across in dealing with the readings on cystitis:

And keep that attitude which has been a part of the entity's whole mental being, mien and manner. Know that the body creates, or will revive itself. Then keep that attitude of optimism and helpfulness to others, and it makes the environment of them the same for self. Worry more about somebody else than you do about youself, and you'll be a lot better off!   **540-11**

ALCOHOLISM

by Winthrop H. Ware, M.D.

Few diseases are as ill-defined and as difficult to treat as alcoholism. Even nowadays there is still a question in the minds of some whether it is a disease or a moral issue. Edgar Cayce called it a disease, and most serious workers in the field today also call it a disease. Noyes and Kolb say, "Alcoholism should be looked upon as a psychic illness rooted in a personality disorder or immaturity." Calling it a disease has the advantage of making it easier for an alcoholic to accept treatment.

Basically, the disease has two phases. First, the susceptible individual is exposed to alcohol and finds that it satisfies his special needs for coping with his environment. Then, when he has imbibed enough alcohol for a sufficient period of time, he becomes addicted, much as one becomes addicted to any other drug. Some would argue that this is an oversimplification, and perhaps it is, as it leaves out all the "other types" of alcoholics, but it will do for the consideration at hand.

If it were possible to determine ahead of time which person had the so-called "fertile soil of addiction" in his nature, then it would perhaps be possible to condition this person against alcohol until he could receive psychiatric aid in eliminating his propensity toward the disease. Studies seem to indicate, however, that it is almost impossible to determine who will become an alcoholic. Thus, prevention from this standpoint must be considered unlikely.

In the book, *Understanding the Alcoholic,* by Howard Clinebell, the author says that danger arises because an individual having heard that "emotionally healthy people don't become alcoholics" will assume that he is not a potential candidate for the illness, and consequently is overconfident. Clinebell further states that there are two points to emphasize in the prevention of alcoholism. One is that an individual doesn't have to be aware of neurosis or emotional instability to become an alcoholic, because many deep psychological problems are hidden from ourselves. In fact, the emotional damage often occurred at a very early age and, he says, this damage has been overlaid by many layers of a comparatively normal personality adjustment. The people who become alcoholics rarely, if ever, are aware that they are neurotic or susceptible to the disease; thus, the way is open for alcohol to reactivate their buried problems.

The second point Clinebell emphasizes is that it is impossible to predict with accuracy just which six people out of any 100 drinkers are potential alcoholics. He says that until such a prediction is possible, we should accept the warning, "You too can be an alcoholic."

Once one becomes an alcoholic, either by habit or addiction, the first thing to do is to stop the use of alcohol. The patient can do this himself, if he has the will power. This is the basis of the AA approach. Or, the patient can receive the aid of a "chemical fence," such as Antabuse (disulfiram). Once an alcoholic ceases to drink, half of his problem is solved. The other half of the problem is the re-education concerning problem approach and solving, as well as the eventual treatment of the underlying psychological problems.

As anyone who has worked with alcoholics knows, getting them to accept a substitute for alcohol is almost impossible until the alcoholic is willing to "try anything." Usually this means that the alcoholic is so desperate that he gives up trying to manipulate people to continue his habit and surrenders to any help he can find. This is called "hitting bottom," and the main work of the professional therapist is in "raising the bottom" of the alcoholic unwilling to seek aid and thus making his desperation come sooner. This must often be done by withdrawing all help and aid from the alcoholic and making him suffer the consequences of his own foolishness.

The difficulty of this task can be realized in the addicted alcoholic who considers alcohol as essential as he once considered food. Added to this problem is the fact that alcohol does possess food value—but no vitamins. An advanced alcoholic suffers concomitant avitaminosis, which leads to cirrhosis of the liver, heart muscle degeneration, destruction of the higher centers of the brain, etc.

In Cayce's work with alcoholics, we note that he had a very shrewd assay of the alcoholic situation. In the following case, we find a young man, aged 31, at the threshold of becoming addicted. Mr. Cayce finds that the effects of alcohol are just becoming evident in his organs. This is what he recommends:

In meeting the needs of the conditions physically, we find—while there must be physical applications for the body to right itself—the greater portion must come through that of self's own will in making for the environs and for the effect that is being produced in the body.   4386-1

He then goes on to prescribe a "chemical fence" to be given once a week to the young man:

Prepare in a capsule, this:
Eucalyptol	1 minim
Rectified Oil of Turp	½ minim
Benzosol	1 minim
Codeine	1/60th grain

This must be given under *physician's* instructions or directions, one each week—until there will be found that there is an alternation in the desires of the body as related to the physical forces, as related to the mental application of self—for this will produce *nausea* to an extent that the body, when over*stimulating* self, will refrain from same. Should this become, under the physician's reactions, such as has been in cases past *with* the body—they, themselves, refrain—or change to such an extent as to increase rather than diminish—take of the parings or the scraping of the fingernail of the body, on the left *little* finger—these prepared in coffee or tea will prevent a reoccurrence. Not injurious, but helpful.

4386-1

Another time, Mr. Cayce prescribed another "chemical fence":

Q-11. Is there anything I can do to help break my husband [1439] from drinking?
A-11. Give him this, and he'll never want to drink any more—it'll make him very sick if he does!
Put into a capsule:
Oil of Eucalyptus	1 minim
Oil of Turp	½ minim
Compound Tincture of Benzoin	½ minim

Give him this.
Q-12. How may it be given?
A-12. In a capsule!
Q-13. Just one?
A-13. Just one. And then he'll vomit his boots up if he takes a drink! The *smell* of liquor will be abhorrent, even! Of course,

he *can* overcome it—but it'll make him sick for the first year
anyway!   845-2

These chemical fences of Mr. Cayce's would seem to act
longer than Antabuse, which has an action of only four days.
The fingernail parings would seem to work as does Flagyl
(metronidrazole) in dampening the desire for alcohol, and
perhaps in the management of a hangover taking "some of the
hair of the dog that bit him."

In the case of a 56-year-old male, we find a more advanced
alcoholic (in the range of the addiction to alcohol). It is
interesting to note that Mr. Cayce found the heart, liver, spleen,
kidneys, and pancreas involved. This merits him a good grade
in modern pathology. He is also quite correct when he says:

Digestion impaired, on account of condition created in
spleen, pancreas and liver. Hence the deterioration, as it were,
of the whole system and the lack of assimilation and of the
digestive system functioning normal.   28-1

In this man, Mr. Cayce recommended both a "chemical
fence" and a certain substitute for alcohol:

Podophyllin	1 grain
Cascara Sagrada	1 grain
Leptandrin	1 grain
Licorice Compound	½ grain

Make these in this quantity in each capsule, making five (5)
capsules. One shall be taken every other day.

Give this as the stimulant and preventative from using
overstimulants:

2 ounces	Tincture Valerian
2 drams	Bromide of Potash
10 grains	Iodide of Potash, with
4 ounces	Elixir Calisaya, and
1 ounce	Elixir Celerina, with the
Extract of Verbena	15 minims.

The carrier for this should be sufficient Peptotol [in another
place he says this is any sweet syrup] to make sixteen (16)
ounces. The dose would be [a] teaspoonful twice each day,
morning and evening. By the time the whole quantity is taken,
we will find the body will be rid of much of the desire for those
properties that overbalance the system.

Should the body take the overstimulus while using this and
become sick and nauseated, use the enema, also the stomach

pump or wash to cleanse the stomach of same, though this would not be a poison in itself, unless there was certain combinations of properties taken in diet. Hence, while these are being taken, the diet should consist chiefly of meats or game, or the juices of same, with only vegetables that grow above ground, and no form or combination of any night-shade variety of vegetable. 28-1

Then, Mr. Cayce gives to the drunkard this advice that almost sounds as if it comes from the AA's Big Book.

Then, for the mental, we find the body very capable, would it only guide itself in the manner in which it understands the knowledge of self. Spiritual understanding only comes from the understanding of the divine within self, and the attempt to correlate same will always bring the development of self mentally and spiritually. For those who call upon the God will not find Him afar off but ever present and ready to answer the self as is found in the inner man. 28-1

Just as important as helping the alcoholic directly is the helping of the spouse of the alcoholic to change her attitude toward him. It is here that Cayce gives some excellent advice. Here is what he says to one woman:

Q-4. Just what should I do about my husband and home?
A-4. As just indicated, live right *self!* Never so act, in *any* manner, in any inclination, that there may ever be an experience of regret within self. Let the moves and the discourteousness, the unkindness, all come from the other. Better to be abased *self* and have the peace within!

For unless changes arise, some great disturbance will come. But if ye so act that these appear to arise from thy neglect or from thy not caring, then the regret would always be with thee.

Then, act ever in the way ye would *like* to be acted toward. No matter *what* others say, or even *do,* do as ye would be done by; and then the peace that has been promised is *indeed* thine own.

Q-5. Is there any chance of his ever overcoming the drinking habit?
A-5. Not if there's given the least excuse for his continuation in same!

But kindness, gentleness and prayer has saved many a soul!
1183-3

What Mr. Cayce is advocating in the above is now known as "surrender." This is when a wife leaves her husband alone and surrenders all concern for him; she does the best she can for herself and her family. Thus by not nagging or berating him, she gives him no excuse for his drinking, and he must bear the consequences himself. Very modern advice indeed!

In another place, Mr. Cayce makes a rather unique suggestion:

Q-6. Can those assisting do anything to prevent the body from indulging in stimulants?

A-6. They can pray like the devil!

And this is not a blasphemous statement, as it may appear—to some. For if there is any busier body, with those influences that have to do with the spirit of indulgence of any nature, than that ye call Satan or the devil, who is it?

Then it behooves those who have the interest of such a body at heart to not only pray for him but *with* him; and in just as earnest, just as sincere, just as continuous a manner as the spirit of *any* indulgence works upon those who have become subject to such influences either through physical, mental or material conditions!

For the *power* of prayer is *not* met even by Satan or the devil himself.

Hence with that attitude of being as persistent as the desire for indulgence, or as persistent as the devil, ye will find ye will bring a strength. But if ye do so doubting, ye are already half lost.

For the *desires* of the body are to do *right!* Then aid those desires in the right direction: for the power of right *exceeds*—ever and always.

Do that, then.

Like the devil himself—*pray!*   1439-2

In summary, it would seem that what Edgar Cayce advocated some 30 years ago is what the foremost workers in the field of alcoholism are just now advocating.

1. The cycle of addition must be broken by ceasing the intake of alcohol. This may be done by building the "chemical fence" with the patient's consent, or the cycle may be broken by placing the patient in an institution. (Mr. Cayce recommended this for some, too.) The patient may find the will to stop, but unless he has a sincere desire, nothing will work.

2. The persons closest to the patient must surrender their concern for him and let him be responsible for his own deeds. It

is "cruel kindness" to support and lie for an alcoholic if this prevents him for "hitting bottom" and seeking aid.

3. The efficacy of real and genuine prayer for a person should not be discounted and should be vigorously indulged in. This not only has a telepathic effect on the usually very sensitive alcoholic, but it has a salutory effect on the suffering spouse.

What Mr. Cayce did not mention, as it was too new, was the importance of using such organizations as the AA. The AA advocates, very much as Mr. Cayce did, a twofold idea of:

1. Stopping the drinking, and
2. Strengthening the will.

The further advantage of the AA is that it helps the alcoholic get rid of his guilt feelings by putting him to work helping other alcoholics, thus performing autotherapy and spreading the good work.

Left unsaid in all this is the possible use of psychotherapy in correcting the basic flaws in the character that make for the "seed bed" of alcoholism. Perhaps in this new decade more and important work will be done in this respect. New centers for alcoholism are needed, and many cities and towns need to revamp their present alcoholic treatment facilities. In the meantime, we must do the most we can to reach those in the grip of this most difficult illness. What Edgar Cayce said about having faith is really most important when one deals with alcoholism.

BIBLIOGRAPHY
1. *Modern Clinical Psychiatry,* Arthur P. Noyles, M.D., and Lawrence C. Kolb, M.D., W.B. Saunders Co., Philadelphia, 1967. p. 178.
2. *Understanding and Counseling the Alcoholic,* Howard J. Clinebell, Jr., Abingdon Press, New York, p. 301.

WHAT IS ADEQUATE THERAPY FOR THE EPILEPTIC?

by William A. McGarey, M.D.

What is adequate therapy for the epileptic? My wife, Gladys, and I have been dealing with this problem for the past four years, and have started more than 25 patients on the Cayce therapy, the first patient being our own son.

The first vital step in this therapy is that the patient be receptive to this type of healing, so it is imperative that the patient be familiar with the information in the readings. Also, we have tried to make both the patients and their families aware of the spiritual, mental and psychological direction they might take to bring about healing.

In the beginning, to deal with this problem, we should ask two basic questions: (1) "What is the nature of the illness that we define as epilepsy?" and (2) "What is the goal of therapy?"

The first question can be constructed in several ways. We can ask, "What are the physical expressions of this disease?" In our present neurological-medical understanding, we categorize them as to the various types, such as *grand mal, petit mal,* Jacksonian type, focal sensory and focal motor. A type called the absence state is similar to the *petit mal* in that one can no longer converse with the patient and his eyes may have a vacant stare.

There is also a type of epilepsy which is evidenced by an abrupt change in mood, such as fear or anger. Other types include temporal lobe seizures, sensory evoked epilepsy, and a nonconvulsive condition which is characterized by abdominal symptoms. (This last is perhaps misnamed epilepsy; when an individual has abnormal EEG changes or abnormal signs in the EEG and has not had a seizure, can we call it epilepsy?) Much has also been written about psychomotor epilepsy, autonomic seizures and *status epilepticus.* Each of these terms, however, merely describes the *physical expression* of the abnormality that produces epilepsy.

In the structural etiology, we try to determine at a research level what causes the discharge of electrical impulses that manifest as a convulsion. It was significant to me that, in the source material I read, 75 per cent of all epilepsy cases are termed either idiopathic or cryptogenic, implying thereby that we actually don't know the causes. Thus, we are dealing with the unknown. In the Edgar Cayce material, there are suggestions as to what may really be etiology of these 75 per cent "idiopathic" cases. The spinal cord and several lymphatic patches are involved in this explanation.

Twenty-five per cent are so-called "acquired"—febrile episodes that have led to subsequent convulsive seizures and attacks, caused by vascular disease, allergic reactions, birth trauma, asphyxia, and so forth. The Cayce readings suggest that detectable brain lesions are not induced locally but are caused by repeated insults to the brain tissue from lymphatic or spinal lesions. In other words, the origin is elsewhere, and it creates a type of reflex—an overloading or flooding of neurological impulses in an uncontrolled manner. This results in a lesion. All of these various acquired lesions, mostly found in the brain, constitute one of the etiologic factors of epilepsy, that is, its structural or physical basis.

Initially, we became aware of the physical expression of the disease, then its structural basis. Now, the Cayce readings provide, I think, a functional understanding. Cayce expresses the idea that the function of a body is to express the spirit, and the bodily structure serves as a vehicle for the Creative Forces in the third dimension.

We should first consider the etiology as Cayce saw it. He said that the karmic influence in epilepsy was usually the basic problem. Karma needs to be understood, and so does the functioning of the life force in the body, which seems to come in through the seven endocrine centers, spreading out as energy into the nervous systems and into the body itself. The karmic result is usually either a spinal lesion or a lacteal lesion, or both. In 37 of the 79 cases on which Cayce gave readings, both types were present. The spinal lesions were not in the spine itself, but in the spinal cord or portions thereof—perhaps the posterior ganglion or the autonomic sympathetic.

Cayce said that the pinpoint areas caused by a spinal lesion also included a lacteal lesion, as in the lymph system, in which there are very small areas where nervous system synapses occur. Thus, when the cerebrospinal system (with the brain as a central control area of our conscious mind) makes contact with the autonomic system, synapse occurs in minute lymphatic pools. In several readings, Cayce explained that the nerve endings in these synaptic points were twisted and tangled, and that this was what needed to be corrected. The condition had been caused by karmic influences so strong that the impulse from them created the tangling.

These spinal and lacteal lesions, then, are actual areas of disturbance, and because they take part in the functioning of the body they are thus part of the causation. Cayce said that within the body is produced an incoordination between the cerebrospinal and the autonomic nervous systems. In terms of body, mind and spirit, these two nervous systems represent the conscious mind and the unconscious mind.

The conscious mind—the brain and our conscious neuro-muscular contact—is involved very closely with the autonomic nervous sytem and its coordination with our every muscular movement. All involuntary activities of the body—the organs, the lungs and their breathing, the heart and its regular beating, the intestinal tract and the peristaltic movements—are under control of the autonomic nervous system; this system has an autonomy apart from the central nervous system.

So there must be contacts in which our conscious mind can establish a habit pattern in our unconscious mind. This unconscious, autonomic nervous system is suggestible; it can be trained. If, however, a lack of proper coordination occurs between these two systems, the conditions—which Cayce described as an incoordination and a lack of the proper coordinations—will in turn produce a fissure between them.

Dr. Walter Pahnke studied 79 cases of epilepsy, and found that a lacteal duct lesion was present in 39 of them. His study suggested a pattern: Disturbances in the lacteal duct area of the spinal segment affected the adrenals and gonads, which, in turn, caused a response in the pineal and pituitary glands.

The mechanism of this set of reactions was not given in detail, and no specific hormonal relationships were described. It was indicated, however, that one way to influence the pineal and pituitary glands was via nerve reflex action and the autonomic nervous system, which would affect centers in the medulla. The readings suggest that these glands have reciprocal relationships with the brain, particularly the autonomic centers. Thus the basic incoordination between the cerebrospinal and the autonomic nervous systems is caused by reflex action from the lacteal ducts, and spinal segment lesions via the nervous system in the glands. The end result of these disturbances was an overflow of neuronal discharge via the central nervous system, causing convulsions in a *grand mal* seizure and the temporary loss of consciousness in a *petit mal* seizure.

So perhaps this is how the endocrine glands are involved. We also have to remember that they are neural-hormone transducers; this means, at least in my language, that they have not only the capacity to produce hormones but also the capacity to originate or receive nerve impulses. Thus, there must be a relationship between the endocrine system and the nerves centered in these glands.

Of the 79 readings for epileptic cases, seven mentioned causes by brain injuries (fewer than 10 per cent). Present medical studies seem to pinpoint this cause in 25 per cent of all cases. But again, this difference in such a small series of cases is perhaps not significant.

Epilepsy might be defined as a functional aberration created by the entity; because the spiritual being has been so distorted (in a sense) in its manifestation, the resultant physical expression is epilepsy. I don't think this is limited to epilepsy, of course; I believe that any disease process of the body must be interpreted in the same manner.

What, then, is the goal of therapy? Should we gear our therapy to the disease or to the individual? I can't remember anyone postulating this question when I was studying medicine. It was never asked because it was assumed we were on the warpath to fight disease. I think, however, that there is a great deal of difference between fighting a disease and bringing healing to a human body. A disease, in reality, has no reality. It is simply a manifestation of the improper functioning of the human body. If we aim our therapy at the human being we can, I think, help that person in a coordination of body, mind, and spirit.

I do not think there is any question that today the traditional therapeutic goal in the treatment of epilepsy is the cessation or the control of seizures. Surgery and drugs are the primary therapies; in addition, psychological adaptation of the patient is often sought. There are also specific therapies in controlling sensory-induced seizures.

For instance, one epileptic patient had a seizure whenever he heard the voice of a certain radio announcer. Eventually, there were three radio announcers whose voices would cause this person to have a seizure. Finally, a sort of audio-immunization process was begun. Other patients were so sensitive to certain music patterns that seizures occurred. Those in another group were light sensitive and, for them, special glasses were made. The glasses, devised in Wisconsin, were electronically controlled so that the light increase or flashing would produce a clicking sound. By concentrating on the clicking, the patient could counteract the imbalance inside his body brought on by the flickering light, and thus stop the seizures.

The philosophy of the Cayce material suggests that the first goal of therapy is the improvement of the coordination of the nervous systems within the body. The second is to re-establish normal nervous system function by restoring or regenerating tangled nerve ends. The third is to bring about the healing of the body. I think this approach deserves a trial by those interested in the Cayce readings.

We should next look for relationships between what Cayce had to say and what is already known in the fields of neurology, physiology, and medicine. We might ask: "Is there any overlapping of the material in the readings with the knowledge that we have from medical laboratories and clinics?"

In the April 21, 1969, issue of *Modern Medicine,* an article by Dr. Walter Alvarez described a form of impotence due to a nonconvulsive form of epilepsy: "For forty years or more I have been noting that some 18% of men who are suffering from a sensory, largely nonconvulsive, and seldom recognized type of epilepsy, have tremendous knee-jerks; and probably as a result of this hyperactiveness, they are troubled by a markedly premature ejaculation. It is so premature that some of the men are impotent, and never marry. Dr. and Mrs. Frederick Gibbs... showed ... that for every epileptic with dysrhythmic electroencephalograms and convulsions, there are ten persons with dysrhythmic electroencephalograms but no (or very few) convulsions."

Epilepsy as a disease is almost always episodic. Many patients experience brief unconscious spells of *petit mal.* They may also black out during moments of great fear, often without knowing what they fear. Some have occasions of violent temper, severe abdominal pains, the shakes or the jerks, brief periods of aphasia or confusion, terrifying nightmares, great depressions, or pains all over the body.

Basically, these are instances of varying emotional responses, in which the personality is disturbed. There are also people who, although not diagnosed as having epilepsy, do, in fact, experience the type of change that we term epilepsy.

How does this relate to the Cayce readings? We know, for instance, that the glands of the body respond to emotions and that these emotions originate from the glandular areas. We know that a person who is given adrenalin has an immediate full-body response that is emotional in nature. We also know that the sex glands, for instance, are involved with the emotions. Thus, Cayce's inference that the glands are vitally involved in epilepsy would seem to correlate with Dr. Alvarez' statements.

Dr. Francis Woidich, in Washington, D.C., has done extensive work in the study of colors, and he offers the following information in his paper, "The Resilient Brain": "We have previously noted the association of red with erotic arousal, hostility, and anxiety. Kinsey, summarizing data from a number of sources, emphasizes the numerous common physiological elements in the sexual syndrome, anger, fear, and epilepsy. Among the data which he cites, the work of an Argentinian neurologist, Dr. Abraham Mosovich, is of special interest. Mosovich has obtained brain wave records from healthy normal couples during sexual intercourse. The recordings obtained at the moment of orgasm bear a striking resemblance to the abnormal 'spike and dome' pattern of *grand mal* epileptics. In view of these facts, one might wonder what could be the therapeutic effects in epileptics of systematic avoidance of 'warm' color stimuli and of deliberate increase of stimuli in the 'cool' part of the spectrum by means of suitably tinted eyeglasses, color therapy, and control of visual environment."

The following reading tells how the sensory system is related to the onset of an epileptic seizure:

When there is an expression or activity from the sympathetic nervous system, or the sensory system that responds through the sympathetic nerve system, we find there is the movement or impulse to and from the brain centers themselves. Then with a lesion or adhesion, the impulse is cut off—or deflected. For, as indicated, we have a lesion in the lacteal duct area, from an injury there in times back; this is [on] the right side, just below the liver area.

Hence we have first an intestinal disturbance through the

activity of the [liver]; at others producing to the pancrean secretions, at others to the activities through the peristaltic movement; not only in the lower intestinal tract but to those activities through the jejunum itself.   1025-2

Eliminations are important in a consideration of epilepsy. In 1895, in an article in the *Journal of the American Medical Association,* a doctor described his experience in the supplementary treatment of epilepsy: "I have traced the cause in many cases to a stomach distended with indigestible food or intestines filled with impacted feces." This observation is valid and is corroborated by the readings. If the lymphatics of the intestines are loaded with toxic substances (which Cayce called "drosses"), the entire body is affected. If there is a reflex mechanism between the lymphatics and the nervous system, there would not be the proper functioning of the nervous system. A person with a low threshold of convulsions would perhaps have a convulsion when this occurs.

In regard to eliminations, Cayce said:

With the activity of the lymph through the area, we find that periodically, when there is the lack of proper eliminations through the alimentary canal, there occurs a reflex to the coordination between sympathetic and cerebrospinal system area; that takes the governing of the impulse, as it were, to the brain reactions; *or* a form of spasmodic reaction that might be called epileptic in its nature.   1980-1

We know that in the autonomic nervous system there is an inner autonomy, and Cayce mentions that when there is a lack of proper elimination, the ability to govern the brain reactions is taken away from some portion of the body, thereby producing a spasmodic response.

Medications by themselves are usually not beneficial to the whole body:

If this is allowed to remain, or if there are the attempts to allay by or through the applications ordinarily in such cases, we will not only continue this reaction but cause greater destructive forces in the areas along the impulses to the sympathetic and cerebrospinal centers in lumbar and coccyx area; thus increasing and making more severe the attacks that occur from this deflection of impulse.   1980-1

Then what therapy is recommended? Here are ten treatments Cayce suggested most often.

1. *Castor oil packs.*

Have sufficient periods of the castor oil packs. To be sure, they are disagreeable, but they will break up lesions as no other administrations will. The best time to take these is the evening, to be sure. These should be given in series; applied for an hour each evening for two or three evenings *before* each osteopathic adjustment is to be made, see? . . .

Keep these up until this coldness *and* the lesion in the right side is removed—which is just a hand's breadth below the point of the rib, or over that area of the ducts.   2153-4

As nearly as I can understand it, these ducts are the Peyer's patches in the small intestines, the largest of which (Cayce said) is an important neurological connection. Apparently, the packs are to be kept over the area to improve the functioning of the Peyer's patches (or the lacteal ducts, as he calls them).

The idea of the treatments, of course, is to correct those subluxations, or tendencies, which exist; deep in some areas, superficial in others, along that area given; but mostly to eradicate—causing the system to assimilate—the tautness, coldness and the lesions in the right side of the body, in the areas indicated.   2153-4

2. *Massage.* Although massage may not be applicable for everyone, in our practice we suggest that massage be given over the abdomen for fifteen minutes and then alongside the spine. This is properly given by massaging from the base of the skull down to the area of the ninth dorsal, and then from the coccyx area up to the ninth dorsal on each side. This is the type of massage that Cayce most consistently described. It brings about a coordination within the autonomic nervous system. The vagus nerve can be influenced through the third cervical outflow or its attachments with the autonomic nervous system; the adrenal can be influenced at the ninth dorsal of the sacral parasympathetic along the fourth lumbar. This brings about a coordination between the cervical parasympathetic, and sacral parasympathetic and the sympathetic within the autonomic nervous system. Massage over the abdomen brings about a better functioning of the lymphatics there.

3. *Manipulation.* Osteopathy and hydrotherapy were frequently recommended in the readings. Manipulation should be given after a series of three treatments with castor oil packs.

4. *Olive oil.* This is given orally (following a series of three

castor oil packs) to improve the functioning of the liver for proper eliminations.

5. *Laxatives and colonics.* Cayce prescribed laxatives, as well as a number of enemas, or colonics. According to the readings, a colonic is the best method for cleansing the internal portions of the body and removing those toxins that may cause trouble.

6. *Diet.* The readings recommended a principally low-fat diet, and definitely prohibited fried foods, pork, fatty meats, and sweet milk. Alkaline-forming foods and vegetables were recommended, but most tuberous vegetables were excluded. Acid-producing foods such as meats, sugars, starches, and condiments were discouraged. In the Circulating File on epilepsy there are suggestions for regulating the diet.

7. *Passion flower fusion.* This non-habit-forming herb compound is not a sedative but does have a calming action on the nervous system. It aids in the eliminations, helps to retard muscular contractions and also has an effect on the sympathetic nervous system, bringing about a lessening of the congestion which accumulates at the base of the brain after seizures. The readings suggest that the reaction comes about to the body from the pyloric end of the stomach as it acts on the lacteals and thus through the glandular system. Cayce states that this substance should be given along with Dilantin, Phenobarb or Mysoline until the latter can be gradually stopped. Then:

. . . the Maypop [used in passion flower fusion] is for the nervous system and for the blood supply, as is hindered by the improper incentives through the connection between the glands at the base of the brain and the hypogastric nerve center, which governs the digestion and the assimilation in portions of the system . . . **4678-1**

8. *Exercise in the open.*

To be sure, the body should take as much physical exercise— and in the open—as is practical each day, not to be overstrenuous. Calisthenics, or *anything* that has to do with the general movements of the body in the open is well. Walking is one of the *best* of exercises . . . **2153-4**

Other forms of exercise, such as swimming, tennis, handball, badminton and others, are also mentioned.

9. *Violet ray.* We have not used the violet ray in our office for therapy, but I believe that there are some cases where it would be helpful.

After these [the passion flower fusion, etc.] have been taken for two to three months, begin then with the violet ray. Especially apply this each day to the base of the brain, or the center or seat of gland, see? Following the whole track, which is down the cerebrospinal system to those glands situated in the lower portion of body, or in and about the [genital] organs. Following the system, however, along the cerebrospinal system, down each side, which rejuvenates, especially, those branches of the sympathetic nerves that connect in their various forms to the various organs as are affected by the sympathetic system, and as are centers for the functioning of the ductless glands, of the reproductive glands, within system.

3790-1

10. *The mental and spiritual attitudes.*

Keep in the mental attitude . . . of being constructive in thought. Not any animosity, nor any feeling sorry for self, or because others are different and are better in any respect enjoying those things that should be a part of thine own. For, in whatever state ye find thyself, or thy brethren either, *that* use to the glory of the Creative Force!   578-13

Let the spiritual attitude be that there is a purposefulness in all of the physical and mental activities, and those purposes not for self-aggrandizement or glorification, nor for preservation of body alone—but rather to the glory of the Creative Forces that are each individual's heritage through the Christ-power in the earth.   715-2

In conclusion, it is our philosophy that all traces of the underlying difficulties must be eliminated, as well as factors which would set up new tendencies in this direction. Therefore, we have decided that we should continue the treatments for six months after the last seizure is reported. We believe that the importance of patience, completeness, continuity, and consistency must always be emphasized, and the aim is complete cure.

MULTIPLE SCLEROSIS

by Ray Bjork, M.D.

Presented to the Third Annual Symposium of the Medical Research Division of the Edgar Cayce Foundation in Phoenix, Arizona, on January 11, 1970.

Multiple sclerosis, commonly called MS, means "many scars." MS is one of the most widespread degenerative diseases of the central nervous system (brain, spinal cord). It is acute or chronic, usually slowly progressive, occasionally remittent. Pathologically, it is characterized by scattered patches of destruction of the fatty covering of the nerves called myelin sheath. Frequently it follows a course of exacerbations (increase in severity of symptoms) and remissions (decrease or abatement of symptoms). Exacerbations may occur at intervals of weeks, months or years. Some have remissions for as long as 25 years.

Some patients rapidly become incapacitated and completely disabled. Average duration of life has been considered to be 10 to 15 years following onset of the disease, but many now live much longer. Often MS is referred to as a disease "scattered in time and space." It is the common crippler of young men and women, usually attacking them in their prime of life. In two-thirds of the cases, it occurs between the ages of 20 and 40. Rarely does it occur before the age of 10 or after 50.

There is a slightly higher incidence among women. Some reports indicate about 60% female patients and 40% male patients. It appears to be more common in northern latitudes, but the reason for this is not understood. No relationship to cold weather has been demonstrated. Prevalence is roughly 40 to 60 per 100,000 in the north in contrast to 10 to 13 per 100,000 in the south. It is estimated that there are 500,000 cases in the United States. Without the myelin sheath, the nerve impulses or body signals go wrong. Destruction of the myelin sheath (demyelination) causes either the complete stoppage of nerve impulses, thus producing paralysis of the parts of the body supplied by these nerves, or impulses pass through the affected nerves so weakened or altered that the parts of the body supplied by these nerves function in disturbed fashion. Scattered destruction of the fatty sheath accounts for the partial impairment of the body functions. Preservation of the nerve fibre (axis cylinder) explains the possibility of remission. When both the fatty sheath and the axis cylinder of a nerve are destroyed, impaired body function becomes permanent. Paralysis occurs late in the disease. Chronicity is a distinguishing feature of the disease.

Scattered throughout the nervous system are areas of myelin. Myelin is a fatty, protective sheath which may be likened to the insulation on electric wire, without which nerve impulses may be short-circuited, resulting in loss of power. The destroyed myelin is replaced by scars which are first soft, then in time become more dense and destructive. The scar at first may only impair the transmission of message from nerve center to muscle. Later the formation of other scars, resulting from subsequent attacks, leads to greater disability. Multiple sclerosis is not a killer, and life expectancy for most patients is not much less than the average. It is the progressive crippling caused by MS that creates personal and social problems.

Victims may be ambulatory, ambulatory with aids (such as a cane, crutches, or leg braces), wheelchair bound, or bedridden— depending on the extent of the nerve damage. Due to the remissions which characterize MS, patients have found it possible to walk again after a long dependency on crutches or wheelchair. Such symptom disappearances are usually temporary, although some experience a stabilization of the disease, a condition which may continue for some time.

In addition to the United States and Canada, Australia and the countries of northern Europe report a high incidence of MS; the incidence is low in the Orient, Africa, northern South America, Carribean and Mediterranean.[1] Sex, race, occupation, urban or rural living are not factors; MS occurs equally in all. It is not a venereal disease and is not contagious. MS is not hereditary. It may be that a predisposition is passed along but until the cause is learned, it won't be known why one of a family is more vulnerable than the other members. More than one case in a family has been known to occur. It is not a mental disease. MS'ers may experience emotional disturbances and personality changes, but these are not necessarily imposed by the disease.

Scientific Research and Etiology of MS

After 100 years of observation and study, researchers still do not know the cause of multiple sclerosis. Many things are dependent upon discovery of the cause: early diagnosis, effective treatment and control, cure and rehabilitation for future victims, arrest and remission of symptoms, rehabilitation. The disease has never in any given patient proved to be the result of a specific cause, nor has the disease, as it exists in man, ever been experimentally reproduced in animals.

There are many theories. Some are based on the similarity of MS to other diseases, some on the response of patients to certain environmental factors, some on examinations of blood, some on affected tissues and cells revealed through autopsies. Some of these hypotheses are:

(1) That a virus or spirochete may be the cause;

(2) That MS has an infectious origin;

(3) That it is due to a metabolic disturbance or defect;

(4) That loss or inactivation of enzymes necessary to myelin formation or replacement is the reason;

(5) That blood clotting, or venule spasm or some imbalance in the blood is the source;

(6) That allergens are to blame;

(7) That some unidentified poison is the agent.

These and others have been probed and reinvestigated. None has been proved. Advances in our knowledge of the geographic distribution of MS may well be a most important and recent development. Observations throughout the world have been reported by researchers in various places. Alfred R. Shotin, Melbourne, Australia, reported a study of the geographic distribution of MS the world over. In this analysis, he suggests the environmental factor. He believes the dietary habits of man seem to correlate with the geography of the disease. He speculates that the susceptibility of MS is the intolerance to gluten (the protein of wheat and other grains) and this may be an inherited characteristic. This hypothesis conforms with criteria laid down by some neurologists and epidemiologists.

This knowledge has held the attention of Dr. Roy L. Swank[2], who directs research at the University of Oregon Medical School and Clinics. These findings have been scrutinized for possible meaning. Experiments to test the suggested significance of these observations have been, and are being, made. If this analysis is correct, the concept of intestinal origin of this perplexing disease may provide a pathway to its solution.

There will be seen a rather interesting correlation between these findings and the statements that Edgar Cayce made relating to the inability of the body to absorb gold; and this, in turn, bringing about the pathology which provides the disease which we call multiple sclerosis. This will be discussed more extensively later on in this report.

Prognosis

The course of MS is variable and may be classified as follows:

(1) In rare cases, a sudden, severe course may lead to death in six to twelve weeks.

(2) In other patients one sees a fairly rapid downhill course, terminating in death in five to ten years. These patients usually have a number of recurrent, rather severe episodes with intervals of relative recovery during the first two years, but are then left with increasing difficulties (following successive periods of worsening), often not living a year or two after becoming bedridden.

(3) In some patients, the course is characterized by relatively minor attacks of brief duration (days, weeks), separated by periods free of symptoms (months, years) and followed by slowly, insidiously progressing disabilities. This may lead, after 10 to 20 years, to some degree of chronic disability, such as weakness in an arm or leg, which may not materially shorten life.

(4) In some patients, the course is characterized by gradually developing loss of the ability to move and a slow, steady downward progression, with fluctuations in the symptoms too slight to be called a relapse or remission. Onset later in life is more apt to be followed by this type of course and, in general, has a poorer prognosis than the remittent type beginning before the age of 25 years.

(5) In infrequent patients, the few widely spaced attacks early in life are never followed by subsequent recurrence or by progressive disability, the disease presumably remaining quiescent throughout the balance of a normal life span.

In general, MS is a disease of the nerves, not of the muscles. However, all muscular activity (contractions, relaxations) are controlled by nerve impulses. Muscles are made stronger and bigger by exercise. Nerve energy is restored by rest. Thus the MS patient has to adjust his daily life so as to do a little standing, a little walking and sitting. It is not good to sit in a chair or lie in bed all the time. After prolonged sitting in a chair or lying in bed, one loses the ability to use his legs. It is most important to conserve energy. The MS'er has none to spare or waste.

Certain factors seem to bring on relapses: (1) poor health, (2) generalized infections, (3) illness with fever, (4) too much exertion or undue fatigue, (5) injuries, (6) allergic diseases, and (7) emotional disturbances (tensions, worries).

At the present time there are no specific agents for the treatment of multiple sclerosis. However, we feel that every MS'er may benefit to some degree from the skillful use of those modalities which are well understood, economical, widely available and encompass a wide range of safety.[3]

In addition to the wide variety of physical therapy techniques which the physician may find at his disposal in caring for the multiple sclerosis patient, a new dimension is added when one looks at some of the concepts of causation and therapy that are spelled out in the readings given on this disease by Edgar Cayce.

Etiology and Mechanism of a Pathologic Physiology Suggested by the Readings

The basic biochemical process stated in a reading for [907] was that MS was the result of a lack of gold that upset the normal balance of metabolism, causing a glandular imbalance which, in turn, resulted in a hormonal deficiency or imbalance. This hormone was said to be necessary for the proper functioning of the nerves.

The reason for lack of gold was tied to a defect in the assimilating system (probably digestive system) which, in turn, was kept in working order by the proper hormonal balance from the glands. (Assimilation involves the transformation of food into living tissue; i.e., constructive metabolism.) Because the glands were, in turn, dependent upon the proper amount of gold in the system, this would lead to a *circular feedback relationship* between *gold, glands, and assimilating system.*

Thus, according to the readings, MS is not caused simply from a lack of gold in the diet, but perhaps from a lack of the capacity of the digestive system to assimilate gold or maybe the inability of the body to use the gold assimilated. In reading 907-1: "Which glands are involved?" The answer was given: "Those about the liver and gall duct."

The only endocrine glands in that anatomical neighborhood are: (1) islets of Langerhans in the pancreas, and possibly (2) the adrenals. Perhaps the lymph nodes around the liver and gall duct are indicated, but no specific hormone-producing function is known for them.

In readings for [1623] and [1031], the liver, pancreas and spleen are mentioned as if they were "glands." The liver was said to enable the other glands to function normally, presumably by the production of a substance which affected the glands. In 1031-2 a thyroid and liver balance was described. In 2564-1 the adrenals were mentioned in regard to the effects of the mental attitude upon them. The readings are not clear as to the exact relation of the liver to the pathologic process in MS. In 907-1 the excretory function of the liver is mentioned as an aid in the assimilation of food in cooperation with the pancreas. This would presumably be the production of bile, which aids in the digestion of fats that are absorbed in the small intestine through the lacteals.

Other readings implied that there were glands within the liver itself. In 5238-1 one lobe of the liver was said to have softened, and in 2997-1 a whitening in the liver was described. Thus, the exact relationship of the liver, glands in the liver, and the other glands remains unclear.

However, the glandular disturbances—which the readings indicated in a general way to be caused by an imbalance between the digestive system and the amount of gold in the body and the liver—were repeatedly described by the readings as a direct link in the malfunctioning of the nervous system in MS. The missing substance from the glands was supposed to be a nutrient to nerve tissue, and the nerves were repeatedly said to lack a proper balance of nerve energy or "stamina."

In 907-1 a lack of nervous energy caused a poison to form in certain nerve cells and then the other surrounding cells were poisoned, resulting in a pulling apart and elongation of originally round cells.

The hormonal lack was said to cause a breakdown of the cellular forces in the nerve walls. This breakdown of nerve "walls" coupled with the description in 907-1 of wasting away or dissolving of the nerves could be taken as a description of the pathological loss of myelin sheath or white matter of MS. There was not a mention of this specific term in the reading. The lack of gray matter was mentioned in 3626-1.

Pathologically, there is damage of both the "white" myelin sheath and "gray" axon in the disease, although demyelination is usually more common and occurs first as the pathology of MS—the lack of myelin is most obvious in the spinal cord and brain.

In summarizing the theory of the etiology and pathologic physiology of MS as presented by Edgar Cayce, it must be said that:

(1) Balance or equilibrium between the organs and systems were emphasized.

(2) Some factors which are not part of the current medical knowledge about the disease were mentioned.

(3) Glandular imbalance caused the lack of hormonal system, which acted to form a poison that, in turn, was responsible for the pathological process in the brain and spinal cord.

(4) The glandular imbalance was caused by a lack of gold and by lack of a substance produced in the liver. All of these factors were to be interrelated by the proper functioning of the assimilative system.

(5) A genetic factor was mentioned.

(6) An infectious agent was explicitly denied.

Treatment

(1) Use of low voltage wet-cell battery carrying the "vibration" of gold to the body.

(2) Massage.

(3) Diet.

"Atomic effect" of gold, as mentioned in the readings, is needed to establish the balance in certain glands that might produce those hormones essential to the maintenance and proper rebuilding of normal nerve tissue. This is not ingested, not injected, but vibratorily applied by the battery, followed by massage. A diet which includes most of the concepts of diet in the readings is suggested.

Treatment for MS has to be of long duration—from three to seven years, usually. Of importance is *completeness, continuity, consistency, hopeful mental attitude by the patient and by those who give the treatments.*

Much of this material has been worked up in a report for the

Association for Research and Enlightenment, Inc., by Walter Pahnke, M.D. I am drawing, to some extent, from his information, which can be found in the Circulating Files.

I am currently working with a number of MS patients as part of the research program of the Edgar Cayce Foundation. Because of the long, extended nature of the disease, no preliminary report can be given, but we can be assured that a beginning has been made researching into this very difficult condition.

FOOTNOTES

[1]McAlpine, D., C.E. Lumsden, and E.D. Acheson. *Multiple Sclerosis.* Baltimore: The Williams and Wilkins Company, 1965.

[2]Swank, R.L. *A Bio-Chemical Basis of Multiple Sclerosis.* American Lecture Series Publication No. 417. Springfield, Illinois: Charles C. Thomas, Pub., 1961.

[3]Alexander, L., A.W. Berkeley, and A.M. Alexander. *Multiple Sclerosis: Prognosis and Treatment,* Gantt, W.H., ed. American Lecture Series Publication No. 405. Springfield, Illinois: Charles C. Thomas, Pub., 1961.

Gastric Cancer

The causation or the factors associated with gastric cancer are dramatically pointed up in a paper entitled "Alimentary Factors in the Epidemiology of Gastric Cancer," by Graham, Schotz, and Martino *(Cancer,* October, 1972). These investigators found, for instance, that those people who had developed gastric cancer more frequently than the controls ate more potatoes, avoided lettuce, ate more irregularly and used cathartics more frequently. Control patients in this series ate a large number of raw vegetables. Low risk of gastric cancer was associated with ingesting raw lettuce, tomatoes, carrots, coleslaw and red cabbage, and the risk declined with increases in the number of these vegetables eaten raw.

Perhaps the most outstanding recommendation in the Cayce readings for those people who had cancer *of any kind* was to move toward a raw vegetable diet, and when a person had a far-advanced cancer, Cayce often suggested that the diet be "that that a cow or a rabbit would eat." The implication from the readings would be that not only are such things as green salads highly important in preventing cancer, but also that they are helpful in treatment.

MINIMAL BRAIN DYSFUNCTION IN CHILDREN

by Ernest F. Pecci, M.D.

From a lecture delivered at the 10th Annual Medical Symposium of the A.R.E. Clinic, Inc., held in Scottsdale, Arizona, January, 1977.

I've talked from time to time in the past about my work with handicapped children. Over the past ten years I've had the opportunity to be a director of a center for handicapped children. Not only could I evaluate intensively some 1500 children, but I was able to follow them every day for several years to note their progress. Also, I have working with me a staff of very highly trained professionals—psychologists, physical therapists, occupational therapists, language therapists and so on—and gradually we developed a very sophisticated team that was able to look at these children in ways that I believe they have never been looked at before.

I've talked in the past about applying some of the Edgar Cayce principles to these children in terms of emotion and attitude. We don't call our approach the Therapeutic Touch, but we do believe in the importance of their being fondled and handled with the proper sentiment, with the feeling that some energy and love is being given to these children, and we think this brought about tremendous therapeutic change in them. We have under our care children several months old; we take all ages, and some of them are the type of children that in the past were automatically relegated to state hospitals—the so-called vegetables. What we found is that if we catch them at an early age, with the proper type of consciousness having been applied to them by other people—love and some other things I'm going to mention later—the changes were so dramatic that the turnover rate has now become fantastic. Although ours is a relatively small center in terms of the number of children we can treat at once, we've seen a great many of them because of the turnover rate. They would actually come to life, so to speak, and they would then go on to other kinds of special schools. It's amazing, the plasticity of the human brain!—its ability to respond to the right kind of stimulation and environment, and a loving kind of setting.

In addition to working with the very severely handicapped, the very severely mentally retarded, we also had a diagnostic center that worked with children who had school problems. These were the so-called minimally brain-damaged children, those with minimal learning problems—children that supposedly had normal or slightly below normal intelligence, but just couldn't make it in the classroom.

I had talked, over the years, with Dr. Bill McGarey, and he recommended the use of castor oil packs. Although I had read about this in the Edgar Cayce material, I wasn't really sold on the idea until I talked to Bill. Several years ago we began to apply castor oil packs to the right side of the child's abdomen, and we began getting some very significant results. We used this treatment with children who were lethargic and sluggish and who had poor complexion, constipation, diarrhea, gastrointestinal problems, and so on; within a matter of days, sometimes, and certainly within weeks, we would begin to see changes. They would begin to brighten up and become more alert; they would adjust to problems and tend to become more balanced. In time we became very intrigued with the castor oil pack, and eventually we were able to get some grant money so that we could do a more detailed study of the use of this pack in combination with other, supplemental therapies that we had developed over the years. One specific area we investigated was nutrition. The feeling that I have is that the pack helps these children to assimilate and digest their food better. Perhaps the pack takes effect through helping the lymphatic flow, as Dr. McGarey postulates. We don't really know how the castor oil pack works, but it does work better than just heating pads, which we've also tried. There's something in the castor oil that in some way penetrates to and stimulates in a healing way the lymphatic system of the circulation of the body. That still would have to be the topic of another research study to find out why the packs work. But as a clinician, I'm only interested in results right now.

I want to explain now a little bit about the point of view we began to develop in looking at handicapped children. One thing

I became impressed with fairly early was that the severity of the organic brain damage, which was well documented—we knew many of them had very severe brain damage—was not related to the functioning of the child. A child with severe cerebral palsy can have close to normal intelligence, as you no doubt know. On the other hand, some children with minimal types of damage were just totally spaced out—they were not amenable to learning. So something else was operating besides the physical intactness of the brain. It seemed an obvious conclusion that the brain, like any organ of the body, needs nutrients and oxygen and the proper supply of energy in order to function, and that perhaps there were some metabolic disturbances.

Now, as we were working with the very severely handicapped, it became obvious that all the conditions that led to brain damage, such as birth trauma or whatever, had associated physical illnesses in the body. These children just were not physically well; they had gastrointestinal disorders, some had cardiac disorders, they had enzyme deficiencies of various types and a number of other kinds of disorders within the body.

One of the disorders I studied more specifically than the others was hypoadrenocorticoidism. The adrenal gland sits upon the kidneys on each side of the body; it's a small gland, and yet we could not survive without it for very long. It handles all of the nonspecific stress in the body. If the body is stressed emotionally or by any of a variety of conditions—like lack of oxygen or eating the wrong foods, which adds to the stress of the body—a good, intact adrenal gland can handle that. So whenever the adrenal gland is really healthy, you have a tremendous reserve. But when it's low and you have this tired feeling, this exhausted feeling, all kinds of disease symptoms come out: you get hypoglycemia, allergies, colds and "flu-like" symptoms; it becomes hard to think; you have poor memory; and so on. This is the result of low adrenal activity.

Now the adrenal gland can become exhausted. Chronic stress of the adrenal gland can lead to a permanent kind of low adrenal activity. But also, many children have had from birth, because of birth trauma or the physiological predisposition of the mother, low adrenal gland activity. So I began to look at the energy level of these children. Instead of asking, "What is the brain power?" or "Where's the brain damage *per se?*" I asked, "What is the energy level? How much energy does this child have to think?" We know that if we are very, very tired, or if we've taken a tranquilizer of some type, like a stiff martini, or if we have an illness or a cold, we are not able to think or to function mentally. If you were in this condition and someone came up to you and said, "Will you read these equations and try to translate this for me?"—or whatever mental task he might ask you to do at that time—you'd be likely to tell him to get lost; you would just not want to think. The brain takes a considerable amount of energy, as you know—40 to 50 percent of the energy in the body of a person who does a lot of thinking. It does take energy to think—a tremendous amount of energy.

So I looked into the energy systems, and together with Doctor Philip Peltzman, a research man from U.C. Medical Center who did electroencephalograms (EEGs) on a research basis with the children, I began to work with children who had no discernible brain damage *per se;* Dr. Peltzman did detailed electrographic studies using a laser beam to analyze the results, and the data was put into computers. And he saw that the average child that is called minimally brain-damaged had absolutely no evidence of brain damage that could be found by any study we can make. Of course, the literature has shown this. In fact, what I discovered was that the term "minimal brain damage"—and this is a fact—is given specifically because there is no sign of brain damage. So they say minimal; if they could find brain damage, they'd just say brain damage. So, by definition, when you say minimal brain damage, nobody's going to be able to detect any brain damage *per se;* yet these children have aphasia (in other words, they hear things and it sounds like a ratchety transistor radio; they can't quite get it—they can't quite synthesize it inside—they hear the words, but they can't make sense out of them) and a number of other kinds of learning problems: they can't perceive the sequence of things; numbers and letters jump about when they try to read; they can't focus; they have problems with poor attention; and so on.

So I began to study the problems of these children in detail, and I got a number of terms which I'll just briefly share with you, because they're rather exciting, and we now train teachers to evaluate children in these terms. We found that the teachers' evaluations of these children based upon these concepts were far more valuable than the professional kind of evaluation, a one-shot deal, that they had been getting by going to diagnostic clinics. Teacher evaluations in our terms were superior to even very detailed clinical studies, because these children change from day to day.

I just want to describe briefly some of the terms we use. We talk about attention span. These children could focus on an object when the object was emitting a flashing light. If the stimulus was in some way striking to the child, the child would be drawn to it. But as far as vigilance goes, or maintaining attention on an object that was not stimulating to them, they were very poor at that. In other words, if I gave you a sheet of paper and told you to look at it, there would be no problem; you could all look at it, right? But if you had to look at it for 30 minutes, you'd have to train yourself in the ways of meditation or whatever to really focus on it for that long. Each of you would be able to focus for a variable length of time, but it would take energy; it would be work to really look at this as if you were a lookout on a ship or a radar viewer. It does take a tremendous amount of energy just to keep vigilant.

On the other hand, if there is any stimulation coming from an object, the child becomes stimulus-bound; he can't break his attention away from it. The tendency to stop being aware of repetitive stimuli is described by a number of terms, such as "habituation." As an illustration, if somebody yells "Boo!" at you, you jump out of your seat; but if he keeps on yelling "Boo!" most people will stop hearing it after a while. Or, a passing train might wake you up the first time it goes by at night, but after a time you won't hear it anymore. Changes such as these are measurable on the EEG, in that eventually the graph stops showing spikes. Now if a child with so-called minimal brain damage is exposed to repeated stimuli like these, he's not going to habituate; he'll become continuously tied to the stimulus, continously stuck to it.

To understand this problem better, let's consider what the EEG can tell us about how the brain works. As you know, the brain is like an electrical cell battery—it has electrical waves. These waves have been classified as alpha, beta, delta, theta, and so on, and they can be changed by various kinds of stimuli external to the person. If you get a strong stimulus, there'll be a spike—an evoked potential, in other words—in the EEG. Now let's say we get an evoked potential by sounding a bell. Then we wait a little while and ring another bell and get another potential. We can show that, after a series of these paired stimuli, conditioning occurs; because when we stop sounding the second bell, there will still be a spike in the average person's

EEG. We ring one bell, then the other bell, and there'll be two spikes; then we do one bell and no second bell, and there's still a second spike.

Now when children are brain damaged, they'll continue to have that second spike much longer than children without the so-called minimal brain damage. Expressing this clinically, we say they don't have extinction. In fact, this is the most singular feature of children who have learning problems—they don't extinguish easily. It's as if they're watching a television set and still seeing the previous moment's picture while looking at a new picture. There is difficulty in getting recent memory, long-term memory, and once they get it, they can't be unconditioned. They are really stuck with whatever they are conditioned with—they don't have extinction. They also have a slow latency period. In other words, the spike may take so many milliseconds to appear in their EEG, whereas in the average person's it may be only a fraction of a millisecond; these children take twice as long before they get the spike. I suspect that this is related to metabolic problems—such as a slow thyroid—or various other kinds of physiological problems.

I'll just mention one or two more characteristics of these children. The first involves the figure ground. To get an idea of how this works, imagine that someone is talking to you and you want to hear something else going on over there; you can sort of mentally block off the one person and hear the other sounds. But doing this takes energy. If you're talking to someone and you want to tune in to another conversation, you can do it for a while; but it's very exhausting, and after a while you become very nervous—probably without knowing why—because it drains your energy very rapidly; but you can do it. We tested this in our children by having a light flash at the same time sounds were being made, and having them try to focus on one or the other. And they had difficulty with this—they couldn't separate. Their brains didn't have the energy for this task. Or if they could do it, it was for only very brief periods of time—not for very long.

The point I want to make is that the human brain—the three-dimensional brain—can focus on only one thing at a time. That's right, you can focus on and understand only one thing at a time. Now, you might think that you can listen to music while you study, or read something while you listen to a lecture, but what you would be doing if you were doing this, or seemed to be doing it, is rapidly shifting your attention back and forth

181

between the two stimuli. Eventually you will find that you're not getting either one very well—you'd probably be getting a lot of confusion. After a while, you'd become very irritable, very exhausted; you can do this for only so long, because it requires mental energy. The same is true of just memorizing rote material. Let's say I were to put four or five numbers on the board·and ask you to memorize them. After a minute I would cover them and come back with some more numbers for you to do. By the time I came to the third or fourth set, you'd all be very resistant, right? You'd probably be very irritable. Because doing this takes energy. Unless you're energized in some way— somehow re-energized and remotivated—you are not going to use your head for thinking, because it's work. It takes a lot of energy.

We found that these difficulties are heightened in the children we're working with. When we had the teachers use check-off scales listing these items, we found that the children had a resistance to learning after a certain period of time, because there's a refractory period to all learning: After spending a certain interval in an intensive learning situation, a person reaches a point of diminishing returns, where he can't learn any more—the brain shuts off and a rest is needed. Our children reached this point very rapidly; they just could not maintain their learning set for very long. And I see this as indicating a lack of total body energy. Even though there was no real evidence that they had brain damage *per se,* they did not have the energy to think or learn. As a matter of fact, children who we knew had brain damage, such as hydrocephalus, or abnormal EEGs were doing considerably better in some areas than our children were. So the problem had to be something other than brain damage.

Where could this energy depletion be coming from? Why didn't these children have a normal amount of energy? Well, we looked at the mothers' histories very carefully, and we found that invariably the mother had had some problem, such as hypoglycemia, at some time, either as a child or during pregnancy; thyroid disturbances of one type or another; allergic tendencies; and swelling or unusually severe nausea during the pregnancy. A number of these symptoms were considered routine at the time and were not really looked at as being unusual. They are the subtle kinds of things that we don't have the laboratory tests to make exciting discoveries about at this point. But when we talked with the mothers at great length, we could see that they had not been comfortable during pregnancy—they had had swelling, edema, or some kind of allergic condition. In fact, I believe that mothers can be allergic to their own babies.

Looking over these 1500 children, we were able to describe a number of syndromes, such as the "unwanted child syndrome." I would like to describe briefly this particular syndrome. In examining a number of adopted children and those who admittedly were unplanned and unwanted by their mothers, we have been fairly consistently able to detect a variety of subtle sensorimotor integration and learning problems that lend evidence to the idea that psychological rejection has a physiological and metabolic impact upon the fetus.

Now it's true that with almost anything you discover in terms of pregnancy complications or health problems in children, you'll find people who had these problems and did well. They had the stamina, they had other things going for them and could overcome the physical difficulties. This doesn't mean that the condition did not impose a great strain upon the body. So some people can have allergies, and when they're feeling really well the allergies are minimal, but at other times the allergies are really overwhelming to them. We found that with some mothers certain conditions tended to run in the families; there was a predisposition to having hyperactive children, children with learning disabilities of various types; there was incoordination in the other members of the family, and more than one child tended to have it. It tended to be more common in the boys than the girls, and I believe this is because females have larger adrenal glands—at least in animals they do—and I think this might have something to do with the extra X chromosome. But certainly women can stand much greater stress than men. Ashley Montague, the anthropologist, has made a great point of this in one of his recent books.

So we began asking, "What are some of the causes of these conditions?" We'd found birth trauma and poor nutrition or other complications during the pregnancy—like the mother having flu or some other illness. But what about events after the pregnancy? We discovered that these children had varying degrees of malnutrition, and this is rather subtle. Although we generally don't expect to find much undernourishment in this country, we really don't have very high standards for nutrition. Children would come to us and we would say, "Wow! Just look at this kid—an obvious case of malnutrition!" But nobody had really been aware of it. They'd just say, for example, that the child wasn't unlike his friends. Also, many of them were eating junk foods—especially sugar, and sugar is poison to children, all children. Just taking children off sugar would bring about a great subjective improvement in a matter of days. It takes four or five days to get this kind of junk food out of the system.

But in addition to this, there are a lot of dead foods being eaten. Processed foods are dead foods, and people who are psychic, who have healing hands, who can feel energy around foods and people, can feel that certain foods—like the food we had on the plane coming over here—is dead food; it has no life at all—there is no nutritional value whatsoever in this food. And most of the foods we are eating now are just dead foods; there's no nutritional value in them. But in order to make these foods look alive, the producers put nitrates and nitrites in them. Or they wash them in a chelating solution to make green peas look green, and in the process they wash out the zinc. There are at least 30 states in the Union that have zinc deficiency as a common problem. Zinc deficiency is so common that if people are depressed, or losing their hair, or troubled by menopausal symptoms, or impotent, you give them zinc and often it's almost like a miracle drug. And there are many other vitamins and minerals that the average person is missing.

Now, a rapidly growing child who is eating junk foods and sugar, has metabolic imbalances, has colic and is not digesting properly—usually he will have diarrhea and other digestive problems—is a sitting duck for having a metabolic system that's going to provide very low energy. He's going to be at the bottom of his reserve. You see, we normally have so much reserve that we can function on our reserve and look normal even under stress, but we tend to fluctuate between an extreme of good days and bad days when we're on the borderline of our reserve. And these children—well, some days these kids are all right and some days they're really bad.

We also learned that hyperactivity in children is not due to an overabundance of energy. On the contrary, when children do not get a good night's sleep, they become hyperactive. And you who have children know that when a child goes on beyond his usual bedtime and gets overtired, he becomes hyperactive; you can't get him to sit down and relax. Hyperactive children have low energy, and just as you can stimulate a tired horse by giving it ritilin, amphetamine or caffeine, we give these children with low energy something to pep them up, and they become tranquilized, because they balance their energies. You may say that this is a contradiction: giving children pep pills and having them relax! But it's not a contradiction at all; they have low, unbalanced energy, irritability, and you give them something that raises their energy level a little bit, and they are able to relax. More precisely, they now have the energy to pay attention. If you want to see if a child is really well put together, just determine whether he can sit still. It's very hard just to sit still and listen, isn't it? It takes a lot more energy not to be hyperactive then to be hyperactive.

Before going into the research proper, I want to mention a little more about allergies—food allergies. It is believed that about 80 percent of the population is under some kind of stress from food allergy, and most of them are not aware of it. Many people have an abnormal reaction to food; perhaps they're absorbing the food antigens from their food and not digesting it properly. The body has to deal with that, and maybe it's doing it automatically, so that these people are not aware of the fact that it's draining them. But this may be causing them to have good days and bad days, depending on the foods that they eat. As early as 1898, a man named Baker described the allergic fatigue syndrome in children: when they're allergic, they're fatigued. And often these allergies are subtle; they don't come out in obvious symptoms, like runny noses. The most suspect foods are cereal grains, dairy products, sugars, eggs, chocolate, potatoes and tomatoes, so we would selectively take some of these kinds of foods out of the diet. Now one characteristic of allergic reactions is that they can interfere with the maturation of tissues—in other words, growth—so a lot of children with these allergies look young, immature, for their age. Immaturity is one of the most common complaints. They often don't maturate at a normal rate.

Another characteristic of allergy is that it can cause edema and swelling, which in turn may create fogginess in the brain— the kind of edema, for example, that women who have menstrual cramps have. It is believed that some severe menstrual problems are due to an allergy to progesterone, or whatever, and the allergy causes this fogginess in thinking and irritability. It can also close off oxygen to brain tissues.

What we also saw in, I'd say, over 90 percent of the children with learning disabilities is that they have very specific problems with sensorimotor integration and coordination. I want to discuss this very briefly. We had to develop new

185

techniques for evaluating this, because these children will pass the usual neurological exam. However, they have a number of subtle kinds of things that we learned over the years to look for and spot, and if five of us were to see the same child independently we would come up with the same conclusions. So it isn't just our imaginations. We base our findings on what may be called "soft signs," because you can't put your finger on them exactly. But we find that they are very significant to us.

Also, allergic reactions usually result in hypothyroidism and hypoadrenocorticoidism. A lot of these children, and even many adults, are said to have low thyroid activity, and they're given two or three grains of thyroid extract without much result. They keep raising the amount of thyroid given, and the problem is due to an allergic reaction within.

I would like to quote a paper written in 1975 by Dr. William Philpott, a psychiatrist in Oklahoma who made a life study of allergy in adults and children. He's doing some very good work with schizophrenics and people in a variety of psychotic states. He says: "Allergic-like reactions can affect any tissue in the body. The central nervous system, the brain, may be the main organ affected, rather than the skin; this is especially true of children. You don't usually get runny noses, watering eyes, itching skin, hives, respiratory symptoms or gastro-intestinal symptoms. Instead you get what is called minimal brain damage. A child's brain is not working right. Moreover, even if a child does have a runny nose, allergic reactions, skin rashes and so on, as he continues to be exposed to the allergy-producing substance, these common symptoms will disappear, so that you'll begin to feel that the child has outgrown his problem. But there'll be a chronic stress to the body, and this will lead to central nervous system symptoms." Philpott says that the infant who is allergic to milk or corn may in later childhood frequently eat dairy or corn products under the assumption that he has outgrown his reactions to these substances, only to develop symptoms like hyperactivity, lethargy, insomnia, short attention span, poor concentration, etc. And if exposure continues, behavior problems can and often do result; these are secondary to the poor learning of social behaviors and arise because of the child's feeling stupid or dumb in a class in which he's not functioning very well.

As I've been looking into this problem I've discovered a number of possibilities, and I want to go into just one more of these. In the literature, it's been fairly uniformly estimated that

15 to 20 percent of the children in our classrooms today have learning problems—15 to 20 percent. What's going on? I mean, there's something really very global going on, and it's not being looked at. There's something wrong with these children. They are getting something toxic, they're not eating well, they're malnourished; something is happening that we should begin to look at. The problem deserves some investigation and effort beyond what we're now doing, which is pretty much limited to defining them as minimally brain-damaged, doing some psychological testing and putting them in special classes.

Let me just give you one of a number of things that can be considered. There's good evidence that a nutritionally deficient state increases or creates allergic reactions. This has to do with the balancing of protein. General health can help offset allergic tendencies, allergic reactions. Researchers have done an experiment which demonstrates that pregnant rats deprived of vitamin B-6 give birth to allergic offspring. B-6 is the precursor to 50 enzymes, and in the face of deficiency of some of these enzymes, allergies develop. Now it is pretty much felt that the majority of the population is marginally deficient in B-6. In fact, it's believed that the nausea and vomiting of pregnancy—this has been studied and pretty well documented—is often due to B-6 deficiency. B-6 can handle the symptoms of nausea and vomiting. It can be given to handle seizures in little children. Now, the contraceptive pill depletes the body of B-6. This should be known by everyone who takes the pill. You should be taking at least 100 to 200 mg. of B-6 a day if you are taking the pill. Mothers who've been on the pill for a prolonged period of time become B-6 deficient; when they have children, the history shows that they have excessive nausea throughout the pregnancy and they get allergic children.

If allergy runs in the family, then the child is a higher risk. In fact, I believe that if other members of the family have certain allergies and one child seems not to have it, the child probably does have it but is showing it in other ways. So what happens is that these children sometimes get a psychiatric diagnosis. When they have this allergic kind of symptom, they often have subnormal adrenal activity, low tolerance of stress, low coping ability—they seem to have low thyroid activity, but it may come out borderline normal. This is the way they present it. They have difficulty concentrating; they fatigue easily; they're hyperirritable; they crave sweets. You know, when you have low energy you've got a sweet tooth, you want sweets, and the more sweets you get the more you want. These children may crave salt, which is even more diagnostic of low adrenal activity. They get frequent colds, muscular pains or various other problems or weaknesses in the muscles, incoordination and allergies. We found that the cerebellum tends to be the most susceptible target organ. Incidentally, the cerebellum won't grow normally if you don't get enough emotional kinds of support, too; this has been shown in monkeys. And so we see children who have poor balance and a number of coordination problems based upon a poorly developed cerebellum, which is due to allergies and/or emotional deprivation.

We wanted to study this in a little more detail, and, within the limits of our grant, we were able to focus upon a limited population. Actually, we were trying to document what we already knew clinically to be true. We got the cooperation of the Valley Elementary School in Concord, where they have several EH (Educationally Handicapped) programs, and we used three of their classrooms for our study. We divided our sample randomly; half of the children would have the castor oil packs and the vitamin regimen and a special diet, and the other half would receive no treatment whatsoever.

I want to mention briefly what the treatments were. The castor oil pack you may all be familiar with, so I'll just go into that briefly. It's a heated pack of flannel soaked in castor oil and placed over the right side of the child's abdomen for one hour before bedtime. It's used about four or five days the first week, three days the following week, and a couple of days the week after that. And the children really like it after they get used to the idea and after the mothers get over their nervousness about the mess and learn how to handle it properly. The children like it and ask for it—it's very soothing. Another attraction of the pack is that, especially if the children get some attention while it's being applied, they get a lot of secondary gain from having it on them. We really have not had many problems with putting this pack on children. And the parents would notice within days the soothing effect of the pack. It's great for balancing the energies, and I think it's balancing energies in some way within these children. Plus I think it does have the secondary effect of helping intestinal absorption, because within a day or two diarrhea and constipation are helped significantly in most of these children. It's quite amazing.

At any rate, we then gave them a proper diet. Now, we did it in a general way; we did not specifically treat these children for a specifically diagnosable condition—we didn't even diagnose this group. We just said, "Let's give them a proper diet and take away the junk food." We put them on a high-protein diet and took them off sugar, jellies, starches and so on. Primarily it was a very basic diet that would be healthful for anyone. In the beginning, certain cereal grains and milk were eliminated, with alternatives being given in their place, though they were reinstated later on. High-protein foods and natural sugars, like those in fruits, were used, and we kept the children away from fried foods, starchy foods and so on. I think starchy foods increase the acidity of the blood, which increases hyperactivity. We also put them on basic antistress vitamins. I found that vitamin C, vitamin E and vitamin B-6, as well as the good multiple vitamins, were the best vitamins to give in terms of helping the adrenal activity and overcoming stress. They were also given zinc and some other minerals, such as calcium.

For the evaluation of the children we used psychological testing, but I felt that the feedback from the parents would be more important. We had a Parent Symptom Inventory, in which the parents listed the symptoms that they had noticed in their children since birth. These symptoms included sleep disturbances, colic, irritability, fevers with unknown causes, and the tendency to get infections. This helped us to pinpoint specific areas that may have been deficient in the child. We had 78 items on the Symptom Inventory. Included in it were a number of behavioral types of items, like "won't listen," "seems to feel no pain," and "is overly sensitive to reprimands." We found a high correlation between parents who noted emotional problems and those who put down physical problems; there was almost a one-to-one correlation—the more physical problems they put down, the more emotional problems they listed. These children were being accused of being disobedient because they couldn't keep themselves still, because they were oversensitive, or because they were overly rambunctious in various ways and developed some pathologic patterns in terms of control.

A lot of these children had other kinds of kinesthetic problems, which involved feeling as well as vision and hearing. For example, they seemed insensitive to deep pain—at times they didn't seem to mind pain; and some were overly susceptible to tickling. And we made a number of these kinds of correlations, involving all of the five senses. What was apparent was that when a person's energy is very low, he becomes oversusceptible to sounds—hearing becomes overly acute. When the adrenal glands are low the sense of smell is increased 100,000 times; so these children go around sniffing and smelling. They have increased smell and increased hearing, but it's not always modulated properly, so they get frightened and put their hands over their ears at times. At other times they seem not to hear, because they can't integrate the sounds.

Like the parents, the teachers were instructed to fill out a rating scale, based on the behavior they noted in the classroom. I'll note some of those items very quickly. "Sluggish mentation": that's very significant; it's as if they can get the answer, but it's sluggish. "Sluggish thinking": that's metabolic, you see. "Resisting change of set": whenever you are doing something, it takes energy to shift activities; these children didn't want to shift—they got irritable and just couldn't shift. And they lacked what we call "cognitive drive." They lacked that drive of curiosity that children should have. We can get children with very severe brain damage that are very curious and want to do things; but these children lack that drive—they don't care about learning, they're not interested. This suggests that something is wrong with their metabolism. These children are easily mentally fatigued. They get caught up with vestibular-sensory activities, spinning and so on. They are easily confused. They're environmentally unaware; it takes them a long while to orient themselves to situations. They have good days and bad days. Their learning is variable; that's very significant. They are hyperactive and easily distracted. We split that type of behavior up into various categories. They are impulsive and lacking internal controls; you see, it takes energy for the ego to apply internal controls—it's much easier to be impulsive. Some of the other items on the symptom inventory are: "low frustration tolerance"; "lack sensory inhibition"; "delayed extinction"; some of the other terms I've listed, like "poor auditory discrimination"; "emotionally labile"—the children tend to giggle a lot or are inappropriately apathetic at times; "explosive"; and "immature for their age."

The teachers were delighted to fill out this inventory, because it seemed as if I were pinpointing their children's problems on just one questionnaire. And, you know, this form proves more valuable to me than a neurological exam. We could pinpoint the various problem areas, and we could also evaluate changes in the children, based upon the teachers' subjective impressions of what they were noting in the classroom.

We did a very detailed fine motor evaluation of these children. And this takes a special kind of expertise that I think can be developed only over a number of years; it takes experience to see subtle abnormalities in motor tone, for example. These children would be hypotonic—flabby of tone; or they would be dystonic—just sort of jerky, with unsteady tone; or hypertonic—their tone was tight, it wasn't being modulated. They would hold their hands in a funny way. This indicates, to our minds, a sensorimotor problem. We developed dozens of these kinds of observations. We could watch a child for even 10 minutes, as he was reaching for a toy or performing some other everyday actions, and our pencils would be going like mad as we'd be picking up all the different deficits this child had, based upon the things we had learned to observe. We also tested them for fatigue—perhaps they could do a certain task fine, but how quickly did they get fatigued from doing it? We also differentiated between fine motor and gross motor problems. We developed techniques to evaluate these children and put them into certain categories: the dispratic kids versus the kids with sensorimotor difficulties versus the kids with right-left midline problems, and so on. I want to add again that as we put the children into these different categories, each member of the team independently would come to the same conclusion, so it was not just whimsy. There were very definite things that we were all seeing in these children.

Now I'd like to get into the results of our study. We had, as I said, the parents of both the test group and the control group fill out a Symptom Inventory, checking off, from the list of 70 items (allergy, colic and so on), any that were applicable in their child's medical history. We found that the two groups were pretty similar; there was no statistically significant difference in the number of items checked by the parents. We did find that out of the total number of symptoms an average of 28 items was checked off by the parents—28 different kinds of things, like sleep disturbance, colic or allergy to food. I hope you understand that there were quite a few items, and any one of you who has a perfectly healthy child would check off a few items. In fact, we found that in a good, healthy population five was the average number checked off, but no parent checked off more than eight in a really healthy-looking population—one in which we couldn't find anything wrong. But in our test populations the average was 28, with a high of 49 and a low of 17 being checked off. So even the very lowest was double what a healthy child's parents would check off in terms of physical problems. It starts to make some sense that there is a correlation here between medical problems and learning problems.

The items that were most commonly checked off were those related to feeding problems: "food intolerances"; "doesn't care to eat"—isn't hungry; "can't stand certain foods"; "craving for sweets"; "finicky eater"; voracious eater—"eating all the time and always hungry, but not gaining weight." The second most frequently noted category was sleep disturbances of various types, and the third was behavior disturbances due to irritability, unpredictability and a low frustration tolerance; these problems made the children resistant to discipline, negativistic, explosive and destructive of toys.

On the side, I was also interested in some other symptoms that were not recorded as often. Many of the parents—up to 50 percent of them in some cases—noted hypersensitivity to sounds and smells, bedwetting until age 8, and accident proneness. But only one of the children in the whole study had a history of seizures. And none had definable brain damage detectable by the EEG studies that Dr. Peltzman did or by any of the neurological exams that they had had previous to the beginning of the school program. Lots of laboratory studies and a great deal of psychological testing had been done within the school, and nothing at all of note had been found.

The teachers' rating scales showed that all the children in both groups had some difficulty, and what they recorded most commonly was poor attention span, as manifested by distractibility or hyperactivity, and we differentiate between the two. We termed a child distractible if, when he was doing something and there was something going on around him, he could not resist being distracted by it—in other words, if he could not focus and keep vigilant on whatever he was doing. This is different from hyperactivity, which is being driven from within to move and push. This is a kind of inner irritability and nervousness that shows up in lability of mood and a wide variation in behavior from one day to the next. You can see a child with this problem come in, and you can say, "Oh, oh, Jimmy's going to have a bad day today." Hyperactivity can cause mood swings, poor memory, a tendency to become easily confused and an inability to relate well with other children.

In general, in talking with the teachers I was made aware that the children of both groups were universally seen as immature, extremely sensitive to criticism, impulsive in behavior and having a decreased refractory period to learning—in other words, they quickly reached the point where the brain turns off and they are unable to learn any more. If you try to push a child beyond that, he will become so negative toward the learning situation that it will be very difficult to engage him the next day. So, when I'm working with teachers in the classroom, I tell them that they have to evaluate that refractory period in the child and not go beyond it; but they should also be careful not to be taken in when the child whimpers or whatever. They have to know, they have to be able to judge him. Well, these children have a very brief refractory period; they can get only so much, and then they've had it— they can't learn any more, and they become hyperactive and distractible.

Then we checked each child's sensorimotor development, using our soft-sign observations. We rated them in 20 different categories, including muscle tone, muscle strength, fatigability, coordination, fine motor control, tactile sensation, kinesthesia, hyperactivity, eye tracking, balancing, sequencing and motor planning. We used a 3-point scale for each item in this evaluation: a rating of 1 indicated no abnormality, 2 showed mild abnormality, and 3 meant the child had obvious problems. Again, we had several therapists evaluate each child, and their evaluations correlated beautifully with one another. We found that all the children in both groups had significant problems in at least three or more of the catgories listed above. In fact, I can say categorically that we almost never—I feel like saying never—see a child with significant learning disabilities who does not also have sensorimotor problems or coordination problems of some type.

Well, let's go into the results. We had a nurse that worked with the parents to see that the proper regimen was adhered to—the proper diet, which the whole family could take, and the vitamins. The diet wasn't really a hardship. Cost-wise, it was less expensive than the junk food diets they had been on. We had money from the A.R.E. that provided vitamins, castor oil packs and the time of Dr. Peltzman, so the parents did not have to pay to participate in this program. Most of the really expensive items—like the equipment, my time and the time of the professional staff—were funded by the County Medical

Services. So a reasonably small grant got us a relatively good study. We are hoping we can follow this through next year with a grant that will provide a little bit more money, so that we can do a bigger study.

After four to five weeks we re-evaluated these children. I want to go through briefly some of the findings we obtained from the re-evaluations. Most of the findings were based on the parents' subjective observations, and these were dramatic. There were no significant changes in the children that were in the control study, in terms of the parents' subjective feelings and the teachers' feelings about changes in the classroom. In the test group, on the other hand, all but two of the children—who had midline problems and showed relatively little change—had very dramatic subjectively measured changes. I'll just give descriptions of a few of them. (Incidentally, we took all of these children off all medication. None of them was on medication during this project.)

A boy, age 12: "Sleep problems much improved, with a concomitant reduction in hyperactivity." Again, I see sleep problems and hyperactivity improving together. Incidentally, what the parents told us made sense, so we could tell whether they were just showing the placebo effect or the effect of enthusiasm over being in the project. This, together with the fact that when something didn't improve they admitted it, suggested that they were being honest in their observations.

A boy, age 9: "Much less hyperactive; less excitable; he talks less; has begun putting on weight." This boy had been eating all the time and not gaining weight. "Less easily fatigued; not tired late afternoons," and so on.

A boy, age 11: "Sleeping pattern improved"—again. "Gaining weight; appears stronger; vision somehow appears improved."

A girl, age 12: "Her spells of dizziness have disappeared; a decrease in her craving for sweets; bed rocking has diminished; her complexion has greatly improved."

A girl, age 11: "Skin color has improved; calmer, less driven; she talks more relatedly."

These children began to relate and talk to other people much better than they had before.

A boy, age 12 (This is after only four weeks of the very general regimen, a nonspecific, general regimen of just good health which every child in the country should be on—probably including the castor oil packs!): "His memory is better;

frustration tolerance improved," and so on. Other similar findings were noted, with the teachers commenting that they were very impressed that the child "can now sit still; he now listens and is less disobedient." Things they had thought were just emotional problems began to disappear. These difficulties had arisen because the child was not able to relate in other ways, and so was reacting out of his own driven nature, his own bad feelings; he had not been feeling good, not been able to concentrate, and he was acting accordingly. As soon as he felt good and alert, he got centered and his behavior became more cooperative, because every child does want to cooperate, every child wants to please if he possibly can. When you get a child who's not cooperative, as a general rule it's because he's given up hope of pleasing or he just can't be pleasing on some expected levels.

On the sensorimotor testing we saw some very definite changes—and again, we had different therapists testing the children, and the results were very consistent. We saw significant changes in the area of tactile sensation. You see, with poor diet, allergies, food additives, toxic reactions, and so on, all of the sensory organs of the body are affected. So the vision is affected somewhat, as are the ears; the children get aphasia, and the kinesthetic sense, smell, everything is affected. So we saw that tactile sensation was much different, and we tested that in a number of ways—feeling coins, feeling feathers, tickling; we used several different tests, and there was a definite improvement. Stereognosis is a test in which you put things in a person's hands behind his back, and you see if he can tell you what's in his hands; these children had been very poor at this before the program, but they became very good at it afterwards.

For some reason, the two children who didn't do so well were those whose primary difficulties were midline problems—they had an imbalance. This is a subtle problem that, incidentally, a lot of children have. People with this condition have trouble with impulses going from one half of the brain to the other. Because they can't effectively cross the brain's midline, the two halves of the body are not well coordinated with each other; the left hand is not really tuned in to the right, they have reading and learning problems, and so on. The two children in our study who had this trouble did not seem to have as many metabolic problems as the others, and they did not seem to benefit as much from the regimen. I felt that having a couple of children who didn't do that well was a good indication of the validity of our study.

On the whole, the control group showed no significant changes on retesting. Incidentally, none of the people who did the testing was made aware of who was in the control group and who was not. It was difficult, perhaps, for us to do a double-blind study as far as the teachers were concerned, because the children in the test group were taking good protein sandwiches and good food to school, while those in the control group were not, so the teachers could guess who was in which group. But, although it wasn't a completely double-blind study, no one was really told or given a list of who was in the control group and who was not.

Detailed psychological testing was done, the results of which were not significant over four weeks. One reason for this was that all of the children in both groups showed such variability. We just do not have sophisticated enough tests to show the week-by-week changes in children, and they do change dramatically week by week. At first we were all very excited, because all of the children in the test group did fantastically better on psychological retesting, but then we found that the children in the control group had also done better. Some of this could have been due to a learning experience regarding how to take these tests. At any rate, there was no significant difference between the two groups.

Let me just summarize. The current literature right now has a great deal of evidence that body chemistry is important to brain functioning. I'm glad to see this, because, you know, I had these feelings seven or eight years ago, and now the literature is starting to show that some of this makes sense. The brain, like any major organ in the body, requires a continuous supply of glucose, oxygen and the optimum amount of amino acids, along with enzymes and hormonal substances to mediate the effective use of these nutrients; this supply is essential in order to meet the energy demands of a new learning situation. So the brain is put to a tremendous stress, and it needs everything that it can possibly have going for it in order to function properly, even when it's totally intact.

Case histories show that the preponderance of children suffering from behavioral disorders and poor school performance have digestive system complaints, sleep problems, a low tolerance of stress, and the inability to modulate their energies. Many of them have mothers who have had similar problems or problems with the pregnancy that show very subtle metabolic imbalances; many have fathers with similar problems. So there's a predisposition, a history of it in the family.

And this study has shown that there is some evidence that a regimen of proper diet, vitamins and castor oil packs did bring about positive changes in the treatment group that were not seen in the controls. In general, there was a calming effect, with reduction in hyperactive behavior and improvement in memory and concentration. The therapy evaluations indicated that treatment improved proprioceptive and kinesthetic behavior, with secondary improvement in muscle tone and fatigability. The psychological testing produced less distinctive results, and it was felt that other tools were needed to assess mild changes in psychological performance over a brief period of time. Similarly, the electroencephalogram was not sufficiently sensitive to record the subtle changes. We hope to be doing more with that in the future, and I believe that, if the study is conducted over a six-month period instead of a four-week period, we'll start seeing electroencephalographic changes in the children in terms of the things that I've mentioned before.

I think that studies like this should motivate us to develop more refined biochemical measures of hormonal, enzymatic and nutritional levels in the blood and urine of children, and to try to reach a deeper understanding of the complex interplay among all of these factors. I believe we should begin to look at our children from a much more expanded point of view, one that takes into account the total person; this new perspective will include not only emotional and physical considerations, but environmental and nutritional ones as well. And this approach fits in very well with the precepts given in the Edgar Cayce readings.

Visualization and Healing

Visualization in the healing of the body is a new addition to medical therapy in the world today. Carl Simonton has been the pioneer in this field with his cancer therapy, using radiation plus meditation. What he calls meditation is perhaps really a technique of utilizing the mind to visualize the healing process in a manner reasonable to the patient while in a mind-state that might be called the alpha or theta state.

During the period of quieting the mind, Simonton has the patients "see" the x-rays doing their work in the body. They are encouraged to create a scene that to them personalizes the manner in which the cancer cells are destroyed and then removed from the scene of action. The therapy is quite a bit more complicated than just this, but these are perhaps most of the essential points.

It occurred to me that this concept must be part of the Cayce material. Yet for years after meeting Carl and being acquainted with his therapy, I could only find the suggestion in the readings that it is not advisable to visualize something which you want. This admonition has to do with things and objectives outside oneself. It was only recently that I came across the readings that I was perhaps hunting for. They point up the importance not only of the patient visualizing the healing of his body and knowing how the therapy is affecting the body—but they bring into focus the loved ones surrounding the afflicted one, and describe how they might be of similar aid in healing the body. The two readings follow, and I think the concept could be utilized with most any disease, if the patient is willing to work at it.

Q-3. Any spiritual advice for this body?

A-3. The body is spiritual in its aspects and in its reaction. If the body will aid self in those applications as may be made for same, *see* self—in the periods when the body enters into the quiet—*healed* as it, the body, *would* be healed. *Vision* self *being* aided by those applications. Know what each application is for, *seeing* that *doing* that within self. Keep the mind in that attitude as makes for *continuity* of forces manifesting through self—a continual flow, see?   326-1

Those vibrations as may be had by the concerted activity of individuals, that may be able to raise their *own* imaginative (if so chosen to be called) forces within self, to see those activities taking place within the active forces of the body, [5576], we will find this will also aid. *Seek* and ye shall find; *knock* and it will be opened! *See* that being accomplished, and it will aid much.   5576-1

INDEX

THE WORK OF EDGAR CAYCE TODAY

The Association for Research and Enlightenment, Inc. (A.R.E.®), is a membership organization founded by Edgar Cayce in 1931.

• 14,256 Cayce readings, the largest body of documented psychic information anywhere in the world, are housed in the A.R.E. Library/Conference Center in Virginia Beach, Virginia. These readings have been indexed under 10,000 different topics and are open to the public.

• An attractive package of membership benefits is available for modest yearly dues. Benefits include: a journal and newsletter; lessons for home study; a lending library through the mail, which offers collections of the actual readings as well as one of the world's best parapsychological book collections, names of doctors or health care professionals in your area.

• As an organization on the leading edge in exciting new fields, A.R.E. presents a selection of publications and seminars by prominent authorities in the fields covered, exploring such areas as parapsychology, dreams, meditation, world religions, holistic health, reincarnation and life after death, and personal growth.

• The unique path to personal growth outlined in the Cayce readings is developed through a worldwide program of study groups. These informal groups meet weekly in private homes.

• A.R.E. maintains a visitors' center where a bookstore, exhibits, classes, a movie, and audiovisual presentations introduce inquirers to concepts from the Cayce readings.

• A.R.E. conducts research into the helpfulness of both the medical and nonmedical readings, often giving members the opportunity to participate in the studies.

For more information and a color brochure, write or phone:

A.R.E., Dept. C., P.O. Box 595
Virginia Beach, VA 23451, (804) 428-3588